CELIAC DISEASE GLUTEN-FREE DIET COOKBOOK

Enjoy Symptoms Relief, Manage Weight, Improve Gut Health for Newly Diagnosed and Beginners

Joe Miller, RD

COPYRIGHT PAGE

Table of Contents

INTRODUCTION

Celiac disease arises when your body's immune system reacts to gluten, a protein present in wheat, barley, and rye. This reaction occurs within the small intestine, damaging its lining and hindering nutrient absorption, a condition known as malabsorption. Symptoms such as diarrhea, fatigue, weight loss, bloating, or anemia often manifest due to this intestinal damage. In children, malabsorption can impede growth and development alongside gastrointestinal issues.

Managing celiac disease involves adhering to a strict gluten-free diet, as there's currently no definitive cure. This inherited autoimmune disorder prompts your immune system to target gluten, causing damage to the mucosa of the small intestine and compromising nutrient absorption. Gluten lurks not only in obvious sources like bread and pasta but also hides in unexpected places such as sauces, soups, and packaged foods, even in beer made from barley or rye.

When individuals with celiac disease consume gluten, their immune system launches an attack on the small intestine's villi, crucial for nutrient absorption. This damage can lead to malnourishment and a range of symptoms, from weakened bones to mood changes and complications like miscarriage.

Celiac disease runs in families, with a 1 in 10 risk for first-degree relatives to develop it. It can emerge at any age following gluten consumption, potentially leading to severe health issues if left untreated. The disease often goes undiagnosed, with symptoms varying widely and affecting more than just the digestive system. Over 2 million Americans have been diagnosed with celiac disease, but many remain unaware of their condition due to its diverse symptomatology and complex diagnostic process.

CHAPTER 1
COMPREHENDING THE
CELIAC/COELIAC DIET

Celiac disease, an autoimmune condition, arises when the body's immune system launches an attack on gluten, a protein found in grains like wheat, barley, and rye. This assault damages the lining of the small intestine, leading to malabsorption of nutrients and a range of digestive and non-digestive symptoms. For those with celiac disease, adhering to a strict gluten-free diet is the only viable option to manage the condition effectively.

Individuals with celiac disease must be vigilant in limiting their gluten intake to avoid serious health consequences. This extends to products that may have been cross-contaminated with gluten during manufacturing or Method, as well as foods containing wheat, barley, rye, or triticale. Given that gluten can be hidden in many food items, following a gluten-free diet requires careful scrutiny of labels and Things To Get.

Thankfully, there are numerous foods and substances that those on a celiac diet can consume safely:

- Fresh produce and fruits

- Poultry and seafood

- Dairy products

- Legumes and nuts

- Gluten-free grains such as rice, quinoa, and maize

- Alternative flours and starches like corn flour, rice flour, and potato starch

- Foods made with gluten-free flours, such as bread and pasta

However, there are also several foods and items to avoid while following a celiac diet:

- Grains containing wheat, barley, rye, and triticale
- Products made from these grains, such as cereal, pasta, bread, and pastries
- Derivatives of gluten-containing cereals, including beer
- Processed sauces and condiments that may contain gluten
- Fried foods, items coated with breadcrumbs or flour, and similar products
- Items that may have been contaminated with gluten during Method or processing

Despite the natural gluten-free status of many foods, it's essential to recognize the potential for contamination during manufacturing or Method. Checking labels of gluten-free products for approval by recognized authorities is crucial to ensure their safety for consumption.

The cornerstone of celiac disease management lies in adhering strictly to a gluten-free diet. Fortunately, individuals with celiac disease can still enjoy a diverse and nutritious diet thanks to the wide array of gluten-free alternatives available.

Incidence of Celiac/Coeliac Disease

Celiac disease is not just a dietary sensitivity; it's an autoimmune condition that wreaks havoc on the delicate lining of the small intestine when gluten-containing foods are consumed. Gluten, a protein abundant in wheat, barley, and rye, triggers the body's immune system to launch an attack on the small intestine, resulting in a cascade of unpleasant symptoms like nausea, vomiting, diarrhea, and even loss of appetite. Left unmanaged, celiac disease can spiral into severe nutritional deficiencies, anemia, and a host of other serious health complications.

The incidence of celiac disease varies significantly both among individuals and across different populations and regions. Globally, it affects approximately 1 in every 100 people, with those of European descent and individuals with a personal or family history of the disease at higher risk. Recent statistics in the United States estimate that about 1 in 141 people are affected, though the true prevalence is challenging to pinpoint due to many cases going undiagnosed or misdiagnosed.

While celiac disease can manifest at any age, it tends to be diagnosed more frequently in individuals between 30 and 70 years old, with women being more susceptible than men. Despite its relatively common occurrence, celiac disease can have profound effects on an individual's health if left untreated or unmanaged.

If you suspect you may have celiac disease or gluten intolerance, it's imperative to seek medical advice. Consulting with a healthcare professional can lead to an accurate diagnosis and help chart a suitable course of treatment and dietary management tailored to your specific needs and circumstances. Don't hesitate to reach out for support and guidance on your journey to better health and well-being.

CHAPTER 2
CAUSES AND RISK FACTORS OF CELIAC/COELIAC DISEASE

Celiac disease is believed to arise from a combination of genetic predisposition and environmental factors, although the precise interplay between the two remains elusive. The development of celiac disease can be influenced by various triggers:

Firstly, there is a significant genetic component to celiac disease, with having a family member afflicted by the condition increasing one's likelihood of acquiring it. This inherited susceptibility stems from alterations in genes governing the body's response to gluten.

Secondly, while genetics play a pivotal role, environmental factors can also contribute to the onset of celiac disease. Exposure to gluten during infancy or an illness that disrupts the balance of gut microbes are examples of environmental triggers.

Celiac disease falls under the umbrella of autoimmune disorders because the body's immune system mistakenly identifies gluten as a threat and launches an attack on its own tissues. Individuals already diagnosed with another autoimmune ailment, such as type 1 diabetes or thyroid disease, are more susceptible to celiac disease.

Malabsorption of nutrients is a common consequence of celiac disease due to damage to the small intestine, leading to deficiencies in iron, calcium, and vitamin D.

Inflammatory bowel disease and microscopic colitis are two gastrointestinal conditions that may elevate the risk of developing celiac disease.

Although celiac disease can affect individuals of any age, it predominantly manifests in adults.

The prevalence of celiac disease is higher among women than men.

Celiac disease can affect individuals of any race or nationality, although it disproportionately affects Europeans.

The etiology and risk factors of celiac disease can vary from person to person. It is imperative to seek medical advice for a proper diagnosis and treatment plan if you suspect you may have celiac disease. Consulting with a healthcare professional can provide personalized guidance tailored to your specific circumstances.

Factors that increase the likelihood of developing celiac/coeliac disease

The consumption of gluten, a protein found in wheat, barley, and rye, triggers the autoimmune condition known as celiac disease, which damages the small intestine. While the exact cause of celiac disease remains unknown, several factors may contribute to an individual's susceptibility to the illness.

Firstly, one's genetic background plays a significant role. Those with a first-degree relative (such as a parent, sibling, or child) who has celiac disease are at an increased risk of developing the condition themselves. Additionally, certain genetic variants can further elevate the likelihood of developing celiac disease, although not everyone carrying these genes will necessarily develop the disease.

Furthermore, individuals who have been diagnosed with other autoimmune disorders, such as type 1 diabetes, autoimmune thyroid disease, or autoimmune liver disease, are more prone to developing celiac disease. Age also plays a role, with the condition being more prevalent among individuals between the ages of 30 and 50, although it can affect people of any age.

Gender differences also exist, with celiac disease being more common among females than males. Moreover, certain underlying medical conditions, such as Down syndrome, Turner syndrome, and Sjogren's syndrome, can increase the likelihood of developing celiac disease.

Additionally, the use of non-steroidal anti-inflammatory drugs (NSAIDs) and other medications may raise the risk of celiac disease.

While possessing these risk factors heightens the likelihood of developing celiac disease, it is not a certainty. However, individuals experiencing symptoms of celiac disease and possessing any of these risk factors should consult their doctor about undergoing testing. Early diagnosis and treatment can significantly reduce the risk of complications for individuals with celiac disease. Therefore, it is crucial for those at risk to remain vigilant and proactive in managing their health.

Possible Issues Arising from Celiac/Coeliac Disease

Malabsorption occurs when damage to the lining of the small intestine impedes the body's ability to properly absorb the nutrients from food. This can lead to a range of health issues, including malnutrition and deficiencies in vital nutrients.

One of the significant consequences of malabsorption, particularly in cases of celiac disease, is the loss of bone density and an increased risk of osteoporosis. Because the body cannot effectively absorb calcium, crucial for bone health, individuals with celiac disease may suffer from weakened bones and a higher susceptibility to fractures.

Furthermore, celiac disease has been associated with the development of anemia, characterized by a deficiency of red blood cells. Symptoms such as fatigue and weakness often accompany this condition, affecting one's overall well-being and quality of life.

In addition to these systemic effects, individuals with celiac disease may also experience dermatitis herpetiformis, a skin disorder marked by a rash, itching, and blistering. This further adds to the discomfort and challenges faced by those living with the condition.

Moreover, celiac disease has implications beyond physical health, affecting fertility and pregnancy outcomes in females. Decreased fertility and an increased risk of miscarriage have been linked to the condition, underscoring the importance of early diagnosis and management.

Another common complication associated with malabsorption is lactose intolerance, resulting from the body's inability to digest lactose, a sugar found in dairy products. Symptoms such as gas, bloating, and diarrhea can significantly impact daily life and dietary choices.

Neurological symptoms also accompany malabsorption disorders, including headaches, numbness, tingling sensations, and issues with coordination and balance. These symptoms can vary in severity and may significantly impair one's quality of life if left untreated.

It is essential to recognize that the manifestation and severity of these consequences vary from person to person. However, seeking medical assistance is crucial if there is a suspicion of celiac disease or any malabsorption disorder, as untreated conditions can lead to long-term health complications.

Fortunately, adopting a gluten-free diet serves as the cornerstone of treatment for celiac disease, effectively alleviating symptoms and preventing further complications. By eliminating gluten-containing foods from their diet, individuals can manage their condition and improve their overall health and well-being.

CHAPTER 3
SYMPTOMS AND DIAGNOSIS OF CELIAC/COELIAC DISEASE

Consuming gluten, a protein found in wheat, barley, and rye, has the potential to trigger a gastrointestinal condition known as celiac disease, which is characterized by an autoimmune response that damages the lining of the small intestine. The manifestations of celiac disease can vary widely among individuals, encompassing a spectrum of symptoms and affecting various bodily systems.

One of the hallmark symptoms of celiac disease is difficulty digesting food, leading to gastrointestinal discomfort such as nausea, vomiting, constipation, diarrhea, and stomach pain. Fatigue is also a prevalent issue, making even simple tasks challenging for individuals with the condition.

Moreover, celiac disease may manifest as dermatitis herpetiformis, a persistent skin rash typically appearing on the elbows, knees, and buttocks. Unintentional weight loss can occur due to malabsorption of nutrients from the damaged small intestine, while iron-deficiency anemia, characterized by lethargy, weakness, and difficulty breathing, is also common.

Joint pain and stiffness may be experienced by some individuals, often misdiagnosed as rheumatoid arthritis, while chronic headaches or migraines are another potential symptom of celiac disease. It's noteworthy that some individuals with celiac disease may not exhibit any symptoms at all, further complicating diagnosis.

Given the diverse array of symptoms associated with celiac disease and the potential overlap with other disorders, seeking medical evaluation is crucial for accurate diagnosis and appropriate management. Diagnosis typically involves blood tests and a biopsy of the small intestine. Treatment primarily revolves around adhering to a strict gluten-free diet, which not only alleviates symptoms but also helps prevent complications associated with the condition.

Celiac disease presents a complex and multifaceted challenge, requiring comprehensive medical evaluation and ongoing dietary management. By raising awareness of its diverse manifestations and the importance of timely diagnosis and treatment, individuals affected by celiac disease can better navigate their health journey and optimize their quality of life.

Overseeing symptoms and addressing complications.

Managing the symptoms and challenges of bipolar disorder requires a multifaceted approach that encompasses medication, counseling, and lifestyle adjustments. Individuals with bipolar disorder may also face increased risk of nutritional deficiencies and other autoimmune disorders, further emphasizing the need for comprehensive management strategies.

First and foremost, medication plays a central role in treating bipolar disorder. Mood stabilizers, antipsychotics, and antidepressants are commonly prescribed to help stabilize mood and manage symptoms. Additionally, supplements such as omega-3 fatty acids may be recommended to support mental health.

Therapeutic interventions like cognitive behavioral therapy (CBT) can be invaluable in equipping individuals with bipolar disorder with coping skills and improving their overall well-being. Addressing stress and interpersonal conflicts, both of which can trigger mood swings, is a key focus of CBT.

Making lifestyle modifications can also aid in managing bipolar disorder and promoting general health. Regular exercise, balanced nutrition, sufficient sleep, avoiding substance abuse, and adopting healthy stress management techniques like yoga and meditation can all contribute to symptom control and overall well-being.

Furthermore, addressing potential deficiencies in vitamin D and omega-3 fatty acids through supplementation may have positive effects on mental health and inflammation, which are areas of concern for individuals with bipolar disorder.

Given the increased risk of developing additional autoimmune disorders like thyroid disease or rheumatoid arthritis, it's crucial for individuals with bipolar disorder to undergo screening and receive appropriate treatment for these conditions as well.

Overall, a personalized treatment plan developed in collaboration with healthcare professionals is essential for effectively managing the symptoms and challenges of bipolar disorder. With the right support, including therapy and access to community resources, individuals with bipolar disorder can lead fulfilling lives.

Tests used to diagnose celiac/coeliac disease.

Celiac disease diagnosis encompasses a range of methods, each serving as a crucial piece in the diagnostic puzzle. The journey toward identifying this condition typically begins with a blood test or an endoscopy, both pivotal tools in unraveling the complexities of celiac disease.

First and foremost, a preliminary step often involves a blood test to gauge the presence of specific antibodies triggered by gluten consumption. When gluten interacts with the immune system, it prompts the production of these antibodies, serving as telltale signs of celiac disease. Among the commonly utilized blood tests for celiac disease include:

- The tissue transglutaminase antibody (tTG-IgA) test, which detects celiac disease-specific antibodies.

- The endomysial antibody (EMA) test, employed to identify antibodies targeting the small intestine when under immune attack.

- The deamidated gliadin peptide (DGP) antibody test, designed to measure antibodies against gluten-derived gliadin.

In certain cases, a doctor may recommend an endoscopy to confirm suspicions raised by blood testing. This procedure entails the insertion of a thin, illuminated tube through the mouth and into the small intestine to extract tissue samples (biopsies) for microscopic examination. Notably, biopsies often reveal characteristic damage to the lining of the small intestine, including flattening or loss of villi, crucial structures aiding in nutrient absorption, commonly observed in individuals with celiac disease.

Occasionally, to further solidify a diagnosis, a doctor might suggest a gluten challenge. This involves reintroducing gluten into the diet for a period, followed by repeat blood tests and/or endoscopy after several weeks to assess for signs of immune response and intestinal damage.

It's paramount to underscore that only healthcare professionals well-versed in celiac disease symptoms and treatment should undertake the diagnostic journey. Additionally, individuals should refrain from adopting a gluten-free diet without consulting their doctor, as doing so could potentially interfere with diagnostic tests and lead to inaccurate conclusions. Open communication with healthcare providers is essential for navigating the complexities of celiac disease diagnosis and ensuring the most accurate and effective treatment plan.

CHAPTER 4
TREATMENT AND OVERSEEING OF CELIAC OR COELIAC CONDITION

Experiencing abdominal discomfort, bloating, diarrhea, and vitamin malabsorption are just a few of the symptoms that can manifest as a result of celiac disease. This condition necessitates the complete avoidance of gluten in one's diet for effective management. Adopting a gluten-free lifestyle involves abstaining from anything containing wheat, barley, or rye, which can be challenging due to the hidden presence of gluten in various foods such as sauces, soups, and condiments. Individuals with celiac disease must remain vigilant about reading food labels and preventing cross-contamination in their kitchens.

Furthermore, the damage to the small intestine caused by celiac disease can hinder the absorption of nutrients, potentially leading to deficiencies. Seeking guidance from a qualified dietitian is essential to ensure adequate intake of essential nutrients like iron, calcium, and B vitamins through proper nutritional supplementation.

Regular follow-up appointments with healthcare providers are crucial for celiac disease patients to address any emerging issues such as nutritional deficiencies, bone loss, or other autoimmune diseases. Additionally, accessing community resources like support groups can provide valuable emotional and practical support by connecting individuals who share similar experiences and exchanging tips on navigating daily life while adhering to a gluten-free diet.

Managing symptoms and addressing complications of celiac disease, such as the skin rash dermatitis herpetiformis, may require the use of medications like corticosteroids or immunosuppressants. To prevent further damage to the small intestine and optimize overall health outcomes, individuals with celiac disease must strictly adhere to the gluten-free diet and collaborate closely with their healthcare providers to develop a personalized treatment plan tailored to their unique needs and circumstances. By prioritizing dietary compliance and proactive medical management, individuals with celiac disease can mitigate symptoms, promote healing, and enhance their quality of life.

The main approach for managing celiac/coeliac disease is a diet devoid of gluten.

Presently, the primary effective therapeutic approach for celiac disease entails adhering to a diet that excludes certain grains. Celiac disease stands as an autoimmune condition wherein the consumption of gluten leads to damage within the small intestine, consequently manifesting in a diverse array of symptoms, including gastrointestinal discomfort, fatigue, and nutritional deficiencies.

The management of celiac disease predominantly revolves around maintaining a gluten-free diet, a regimen that must be followed indefinitely. This involves the elimination of all wheat, barley, and rye products such as bread, pasta, cereal, and baked goods. Notably, oats can also harbor gluten contamination during processing, necessitating avoidance for individuals with celiac disease.

Numerous commonplace foods and Things To Get contain gluten, and inadvertent gluten exposure can occur during meal Method. Nevertheless, with careful consideration and informed decision-making, a well-constructed gluten-free diet can be sustained.

Individuals with celiac disease who adopt a gluten-free diet often experience remarkable reductions in their symptoms and intestinal damage. Moreover, individuals with non-celiac gluten sensitivity, experiencing symptoms akin to celiac disease upon gluten ingestion but without the same immunological response or intestinal damage, may also find relief from adhering to a gluten-free diet.

While a gluten-free diet can offer substantial benefits for those with celiac disease, it may not be the optimal choice for everyone. Without a medical rationale, eliminating gluten from the diet could result in nutritional deficiencies and other health complications. Furthermore, individuals with specific medical conditions or dietary constraints may find it challenging to adhere to a gluten-free diet.

For individuals suspecting they may have celiac disease or gluten sensitivity, consulting a physician or trained dietitian is paramount. They can assist in formulating an appropriate treatment plan and ensure that nutritional needs are adequately met.

CHAPTER 5
DIETARY ASPECTS TO CONSIDER FOR THOSE ON A CELIAC/COELIAC DIET

If you've chosen to embrace a gluten-free lifestyle to manage celiac disease, it's crucial to ensure you're meeting all of your body's nutritional needs. Here are some key points to consider as you navigate a celiac-friendly diet:

First and foremost, adhering to a gluten-free diet means steering clear of foods containing wheat, barley, or rye. This necessitates substituting gluten-containing grains with alternatives like quinoa, rice, and maize.

While whole grains are an excellent source of fiber, it's essential to monitor your intake carefully. Gluten-free whole grains such as quinoa and brown rice, along with fruits, vegetables, nuts, and other naturally gluten-free foods, can all contribute to your daily fiber intake.

Iron deficiency anemia is a common concern for individuals with celiac disease due to potential malabsorption issues. Foods rich in iron, such as red meat, chicken, fish, beans, and iron-fortified cereals, are all recommended sources. If you're not getting enough iron from your diet, your healthcare provider may suggest an iron supplement.

Given the increased risk of osteoporosis associated with celiac disease, adequate calcium and vitamin D intake is essential. Dairy products, leafy greens, and fortified foods like tofu and orange juice are excellent calcium sources, while vitamin D is naturally present in milk, morning cereals, and other fortified foods. Fatty fish and egg yolks also offer valuable sources of these nutrients. If you struggle to obtain enough calcium and vitamin D from your diet, supplementation may be necessary.

People with celiac disease may also experience challenges absorbing other B vitamins, such as folate and vitamin B12. Fortunately, foods like beans, citrus fruits, and greens are rich in folate, while vitamin B12 is primarily found in animal-derived foods such as meat, fish, and dairy. Inadequate dietary intake of B vitamins may warrant supplementation.

Zinc absorption may also be compromised in individuals with celiac disease. Foods such as red meat, chicken, shellfish, and fortified breakfast cereals can help boost zinc levels in the body.

For personalized nutritional guidance, consulting a licensed dietitian can be immensely beneficial. A dietitian can help you develop a tailored nutrition plan, advise on appropriate dietary supplements, and recommend meals rich in essential nutrients. It's also essential to carefully scrutinize food labels and opt for fortified gluten-free products whenever possible, as many options are now available.

By paying close attention to your dietary choices and ensuring you're meeting your body's nutritional requirements, you can effectively manage celiac disease and support your overall health and well-being.

Dietary Options Suitable for a Celiac/Coeliac Diet

Celiacs and coeliacs must eliminate wheat, barley, and rye from their diets since these grains contain gluten. However, the diet may still contain many delicious and healthy options. Here are some gluten-free options for those with celiac disease or gluten sensitivity:

Gluten-free grains and starches

There exists a plethora of nutritious substitutes for grains and starches devoid of gluten, which can be seamlessly integrated into a well-rounded dietary regimen. Let's delve into a comprehensive exploration of these alternatives:

Rice : An incredibly versatile and gluten-free grain, rice can be employed in an array of culinary delights, ranging from stir-fries to casseroles and pilafs. Notably, brown rice stands out for its rich mineral content and fiber, rendering it an optimal choice for health-conscious individuals.

Corn : Another staple gluten-free grain, corn manifests in various forms, from tortillas and chips to bread and polenta. Noteworthy for its antioxidant properties and dietary fiber content, corn serves as a wholesome addition to any meal.

Potatoes : Renowned for their versatility, potatoes grace numerous cuisines worldwide, featuring in dishes like mashed potatoes, roasted potatoes, and potato salad. Naturally gluten-free, they offer a plentiful supply of vitamin C, potassium, and fiber.

Quinoa : A favored choice among vegans and vegetarians, quinoa emerges as a protein and fiber powerhouse. Ideal for inclusion in soups, salads, and bowls, this gluten-free grain adds both nutrition and flavor to diverse culinary creations.

Buckwheat : Despite its deceptive name, buckwheat contains no gluten whatsoever. Packed with nutrients, it lends itself well to dishes like pancakes, cereal, and even soba noodles, offering a healthy twist to traditional recipes.

Sorghum : High in fiber and antioxidants, sorghum boasts a mild, nutty flavor that complements a myriad of dishes, from salads and soups to oatmeal and pilafs.

Millet : Abundant in fiber and B vitamins, millet serves as a gluten-free grain suitable for dishes like oatmeal, pilaf, and salads, adding both nutritional value and texture.

It's imperative to exercise caution when purchasing gluten-free grains and starches, ensuring they originate from facilities devoid of wheat, barley, or rye to prevent cross-contamination. Additionally, individuals can explore a wide array of gluten-free flours and baking Things To Get, such as almond flour, coconut flour, and tapioca starch, as viable substitutes in recipes.

Moving beyond grains and starches, fruits and vegetables emerge as invaluable components of a gluten-free diet, brimming with essential vitamins, minerals, and fiber. From antioxidant-rich berries to citrus fruits bursting with vitamin C, and from potassium-packed bananas to fiber-rich apples, the options are endless.

Leafy greens like spinach, kale, and collard greens offer crucial nutrients without any gluten, while cruciferous vegetables such as broccoli, cauliflower, and Brussels sprouts further enrich the diet with their nutritional bounty.

However, meticulous attention should be paid to washing fruits and vegetables thoroughly to eliminate any traces of dirt or potential sources of gluten cross-contamination. Moreover, processed fruits in syrup or vegetables in sauces should be avoided to mitigate the risk of inadvertent gluten exposure.

Whole, unprocessed foods like fruits and vegetables serve as the cornerstone of a gluten-free diet, offering a myriad of health benefits while minimizing the risk of gluten contamination from processed foods and sauces. By incorporating a diverse array of fruits and vegetables into their diet, individuals with celiac/coeliac disease can effectively manage their condition and enhance overall health and well-being.

Moving on to protein sources, individuals with celiac/coeliac disease must have access to gluten-free alternatives to meet their nutritional needs adequately. Fresh cuts of lean meat and poultry, along with fresh fish and seafood, offer excellent sources of protein without any gluten.

Legumes like lentils, chickpeas, and black beans stand out as protein-rich alternatives suitable for salads, stews, and various hot or cold dishes. Nuts and seeds, including almonds, cashews, chia seeds, and sunflower seeds, provide not only protein but also healthy fats, making them ideal additions to salads or standalone snacks.

Dairy products like milk, cheese, and yogurt offer ample protein, but individuals with lactose intolerance may opt for lactose-free dairy products or plant-based milk alternatives like almond milk, soy milk, or rice milk. It's crucial to choose fortified non-dairy milk to ensure an adequate intake of essential nutrients like calcium and vitamin D.

Eggs serve as a versatile protein source suitable for various culinary Methods, while whey, pea, and soy protein powders offer convenient options for boosting protein intake, especially for those with busy lifestyles.

To ensure adequate protein intake while adhering to a gluten-free diet, consulting with a healthcare professional or registered dietitian is advisable. They can provide personalized guidance to ensure individuals meet their nutritional requirements while maintaining a healthy diet.

Moving on to dairy products and alternatives, some individuals with celiac disease may also have lactose intolerance or dairy allergies, necessitating the exploration of suitable substitutes. Lactose-free dairy products offer a viable alternative for those with lactose intolerance, including lactose-free milk, yogurt, and cheese.

Plant-based milk alternatives like almond milk, soy milk, and rice milk cater to individuals with lactose intolerance or dairy allergies, providing a rich source of calcium and vitamin D. However

, it's essential to opt for fortified varieties to ensure adequate nutrient intake.

For those seeking dairy-free cheese alternatives, options such as nut-based cheeses, soy-based cheeses, and coconut-based cheeses offer flavorful substitutes suitable for various culinary applications. Additionally, nutritional yeast serves as a savory seasoning option that imparts a cheesy flavor to dishes without any dairy or gluten.

Individuals adhering to a gluten-free diet can explore a plethora of dairy products and alternatives to meet their nutritional needs while accommodating any dietary restrictions or allergies they may have. By incorporating a diverse array of lactose-free dairy products, plant-based milk alternatives, and dairy-free cheese substitutes into their diet, individuals can enjoy a nutritious and flavorful eating experience while managing their celiac disease effectively.

Foods that are not recommended on a Celiac/Coeliac Diet.

Celiac disease and gluten sensitivity pose significant dietary challenges for individuals, necessitating the adoption of a gluten-free lifestyle to manage their conditions effectively and alleviate symptoms. Gluten, a protein found in wheat, barley, and rye, as well as in various other grains and processed foods, can trigger adverse reactions in those with celiac disease or gluten sensitivity.

A celiac or gluten-sensitive diet involves the exclusion of several key food items:

- Wheat, encompassing all its derivatives from flour to bran to germ to starch, is commonly found in staple foods such as bread, pasta, cereal, and pastries.

- Barley, frequently used in brewing beer and preparing stews, is also present in products like barley vinegar, malt, and malt flour.

- Rye, another wheat variant commonly used in baking, is found in rye flour and rye whiskey.

- Additional grains such as spelt, kamut, and farro may also contain gluten.

Furthermore, hidden sources of gluten can lurk in many processed foods that are commonly consumed, including deli meats, canned soups, and salad dressings. Therefore, it is essential to meticulously check ingredient lists before purchasing any product to ensure it does not contain wheat, barley, or rye.

Moreover, condiments and sauces like soy sauce, hoisin sauce, and Worcestershire sauce can also contain gluten. It is crucial to opt for gluten-free alternatives or prepare homemade versions to avoid inadvertent gluten consumption.

While beer is often brewed using barley, resulting in gluten presence, there are gluten-free beer options available for those adhering to a gluten-free diet.

Although oats themselves may not inherently contain gluten, they are often processed in facilities that also handle wheat, barley, and rye. Consequently, individuals with celiac disease or gluten sensitivity may need to avoid oats altogether or select oats that have been certified as gluten-free.

Fortunately, there are numerous naturally gluten-free foods, including fruits, vegetables, meats, and dairy products, which can form the foundation of a celiac or gluten-sensitive diet. Additionally, it is essential to scrutinize processed meals and sauces diligently to ensure they do not contain gluten, emphasizing the importance of thorough label reading.

By adhering to a gluten-free diet, individuals with celiac disease or gluten sensitivity can effectively manage their condition and prevent symptoms from manifesting, enabling them to lead healthier and more comfortable lives.

BREAKFAST RECIPES FOR A CELIAC DIET

Protein-Packed Breakfast Bars

Things To Get

for 24 bars

BASE

- ¼ cup flax meal(40 g)

- ¾ cup water(180 mL)

- 6 cups rolled oats(540 g)

- 6 cups quinoa(1 kg), cooked

- 4 teaspoons baking powder

- 1 teaspoon salt

- 1 cup maple syrup(220 g)

- ½ cup refined coconut oil(120 mL), melted

- 2 teaspoons vanilla extract

- 4 ripe bananas, mashed

FILLINGS

PEANUT BUTTER CHOCOLATE CHIP

- 6 tablespoons peanut butter

- 5 tablespoons mini chocolate chips

APPLE CINNAMON

- ¾ cup gala apple(90 g), diced

- 6 tablespoons walnuts, chopped

- 1 ½ tablespoons cinnamon

- ¼ teaspoon nutmeg

CARROT CAKE

- ¾ cup carrot(30 g), grated

- 3 teaspoons cinnamon

- ¼ teaspoon nutmeg

- 3 tablespoons almond butter

MIXED BERRY

- 3 tablespoons almond butter

- ⅓ cup Strawberries(55 g), diced

- ⅓ cup raspberries(40 g)

- ⅓ cup blueberries(40 g)

- nonstick cooking spray

Method

1. Preheat the oven to 375°F (190°C).

2. To make the flax eggs, combine the flax meal and water in a small bowl and mix well. Set aside for 10 minutes to gel.

3. In a large bowl, combine the oats, quinoa, baking powder, salt, maple syrup, coconut oil, vanilla, flax eggs, and bananas, and mix until well-combined.

4. Divide the base dough equally between 4 medium bowls.

5. Add the peanut butter and chocolate chips to 1 bowl and mix until combined.

6. Add the apple, walnuts, cinnamon, and nutmeg to another bowl and mix until combined.

7. Add the carrots, cinnamon, nutmeg, and almond butter to another bowl and mix until combined.

8. Add the almond butter, strawberries, raspberries, and blueberries to the last bowl and mix until combined.

9. Grease 2 9x13-inch (23x33-cm) baking pans with nonstick spray. Transfer the bar mixtures to the pans, packing each mixture into half of a pan with a spoon or spatula.

10. Bake for 25-30 minutes, until the edges are slightly golden brown.

11. Remove the pans from the oven and let the bars cool for 20 minutes, then refrigerate for at least 30 minutes, or up to 5 days. Gently cut each flavor into 6 bars, then remove from the pans with a spatula.

12. Enjoy!

Pesto Chicken Low-carb Broccoli Parmesan Cups

Things To Get

for 12 servings

- 2 cups broccoli floret(300 g)

- 1 clove garlic, minced

- 1 cup grated parmesan cheese(110 g)

- 1 egg

- 2 tablespoons olive oil, divided

- 2 boneless, skinless chicken breasts, cubed

- salt, to taste

- pepper, to taste

- 1 cup pesto(230 g)

- 1 ½ cups cherry tomato(300 g), halved

• 1 tablespoon fresh basil, chopped

Method

1. Preheat oven to 375°F (190°C).

2. In a food processor add the broccoli, Parmesan, 1 clove of garlic, 1egg and 1 tablespoon of olive oil. Pulse until mixture forms a dough like texture, about 2 minutes.

3. Place 1 tablespoon of the broccoli mixture and press into a well greased muffin tin. Form the mixture into a cup, making the bottom and sides ½-inches (1 cm) thick.

4. Bake for about 30 minutes until the edges are golden and crispy and the bottom is firm.

5. Cool the broccoli cups. Once cooled, remove from the muffin tin.

6. Heat 1 tablespoon olive oil in a large skillet medium heat. Add the chicken and season with salt and pepper, and cook until golden on all sides.

7. Add the pesto and stir to combine. Remove from the heat.

8. Fill the broccoli Parmesan cups with the pesto chicken. Top with slices of tomatoes and basil.

9. Broccoli Parmesan Cups can be stored up to 3 days and can be reheated in the oven.

10. Enjoy!

Jalapeno Jelly

Things To Get

for 7 half-pint jars

- 12 oz jalapeño pepper(340 g), (about 12 med)

- 2 cups cider vinegar(480 mL), divided

- 6 cups sugar(1.2 kg)

- 2 pouches Ball® RealFruit™ Liquid Pectin

Method

1. Prepare boiling water canner. Heat jars in simmering water until ready for use. Do not boil. Wash lids in warm soapy water and set bands aside.

2. Purée peppers in food processor or blender with 1 cup (240 ml) cider vinegar until smooth. Do not strain purée.

3. Combine purée with remaining 1 cup (240 ml) cider vinegar and sugar. Bring to a boil

over high heat. Boil 10 minutes, stirring frequently.

4. Add Ball® RealFruit™ Liquid Pectin, immediately squeezing entire contents from pouches. Continue to boil hard for 1 minute, stirring constantly. Remove from heat. Skim foam if necessary.

5. Ladle hot jalapeño jelly into hot jars leaving ¼ inch (6 mm) headspace. Wipe rim. Center lid on jar. Apply band until fit is fingertip tight.

6. Process in a boiling water canner for 10 minutes, adjusting for altitude. Remove jars and cool. Check lids for seal after 24 hours. Lid should not flex up and down when center is pressed.

7. Enjoy!

Peach Low Sugar Jam

Things To Get

for 5 (8-ounce) half-pint jars

- 2 ¼ lb crushed ripe peaches(1 kg), 7 medium peaches

- ⅓ cup water(80 mL)

- 2 tablespoons lemon juice, bottled

- 1 cup sugar(200 g)

- 3 tablespoons Ball® RealFruit™ Low or No-Sugar Needed Pectin

Method

1. Prepare boiling water canner. Heat jars in simmering water until ready to use. Do not boil. Wash lids in warm soapy water and set aside with bands.

2. Combine crushed peaches, water, lemon juice, and sugar in a medium saucepan. Gradually stir in Ball® RealFruit™ Low or No-Sugar Needed Pectin. Bring mixture to a full rolling boil that cannot be stirred down. Boil hard for 1 minute, stirring constantly. Remove from heat. Skim foam if necessary.

3. Ladle hot jam into a hot jar leaving a ¼-inch headspace. Remove air bubbles. Wipe jar rim. Center lid on jar and apply band. Adjust to fingertip tight. Place jar in boiling water canner. Repeat until all jars are filled.

4. Process jars 10 minutes, adjusting for altitude. Turn off heat, remove lid, then let jars stand 5 minutes. Remove jars and cool 12–24 hours. Check lids for seal. They should not flex when center is pressed.

5. Enjoy!

Easy Gluten Free Oatmeal Pancake

Things To Get

for 2 servings

- 200 g rolled oats(200 g)

- ½ teaspoon nutmeg

- 1 teaspoon cinnamon

- 2 teaspoons baking powder

- ½ teaspoon salt

- 2 cups almond milk(240 mL), (or milk of your choice)

- 2 eggs

Method

1. Add the rolled oats to a blender and blend till they resemble a flour-like consistency. Then, spoon them into a bowl.

2. Also to the bowl, add in the baking powder, salt, cinnamon and nutmeg and mix with a spoon. Then, add in the milk and eggs and mix till well incorporated. Set mixture aside for 5-8 minutes to thicken up.

3. While waiting, place a pan over a low-medium flame and let it warm.

4. When pancake mixture is thickened, grease pan with vegan butter and ladle 2-3 tablespoonfuls of mix onto pan. Cook 2-3 minutes on each side, until golden.

5. Serve pancakes with whipped cream, maple syrup or jam, and raspberries.

6. *Note:* If you are using store bought oat flour - approximately 1.75 cups of oat flour = 1 cup of rolled oats.

7. Enjoy!

Whipped Coffee

Things To Get

for 1 serving

- 2 tablespoons hot water(28 g)

- 2 tablespoons sugar(24 g)

- 2 tablespoons instant coffee powder(12 g)

- milk, to serve

- ice, to serve

Method

1. Add the hot water, sugar, and instant coffee to a bowl.

2. Either hand whisk or use an electric mixer until the mixture is fluffy and light.

3. To serve, spoon a dollop over a cup of milk with ice in it and stir.

4. Enjoy!

Grain-Free Honey Almond Cinnamon Muffins

Things To Get

for 9 muffins

- 2 ½ cups blanched almond flour

- ½ teaspoon salt

- 1 tablespoon cinnamon

- 2 teaspoons baking powder

- ½ cup honey

- 1 teaspoon vanilla extract

- ¼ teaspoon almond extract, or 1/2 teaspoon, optional

- 5 tablespoons melted butter

- 3 large eggs, beaten

Method

1. Preheat oven to 375°F (190°C), and put paper liners in 9 standard-sized muffin cups (you may end up with a bit more).

2. Combine the almond flour, salt, cinnamon, and baking powder.

3. In a larger bowl, whisk together the honey, vanilla and almond extracts, melted butter, and eggs.

4. Blend the wet and dry Things To Get well, then divide among muffin cups.

5. Bake for 20-25 minutes, or until browning and just done (moist crumbs on a toothpick are okay).

Coconut Yogurt

Things To Get

for 4 servings

• 1 can full-fat coconut milk

- 2 vegan probiotic capsules, minimum 50 billion CFUs

- mix in of choice

Method

1. Transfer the coconut milk to a clean 16-ounce (455 G) glass jar. 1 at a time, open the probiotic capsules and pour the powder into the coconut milk, stirring well with a non-metal utensil after each addition to evenly distribute.

2. Loosely cover the jar with cheesecloth and secure with a rubber band or kitchen twine. Leave the yogurt to ferment in a cool, dark place for at least 12 hours, up to 24 hours. The longer it ferments, the tangier the yogurt will be.

3. Stir in any mix-ins of your choosing.

4. Transfer the yogurt to the refrigerator to cool completely, about 2 hours. Store in the fridge for up to 1 week.

5. Enjoy!

Gluten-Free Cauliflower Toast

Things To Get

for 2 servings

- 1 large egg

- 2 tablespoons flax meal

- 2 cups riced cauliflower(400 g)

- 1 ½ cups almond meal(225 g)

- 1 ½ teaspoons garlic powder

- 1 teaspoon onion powder

- 1 ½ teaspoons kosher salt

- 2 teaspoons canola oil

- nonstick cooking spray, for greasing

- topping of your choice, for serving

SPECIAL EQUIPMENT

- cast iron pan, 4 1/2 in (11 cm)

Method

1. Preheat the oven to 350°F (180°C).

2. In a small bowl, whisk together the egg and flax meal. Let sit for at least 5 minutes to gel.

3. In a medium microwave-safe bowl, microwave the riced cauliflower for 3-4 minutes on medium power until steamed and mashable with a fork. Let cool for 5 minutes, or until safe to handle.

4. Transfer the cauliflower to a clean kitchen towel and wring out all of the moisture. You should be left with about 1½ cups (450 G) of cauliflower.

5. In a food processor, combine the cauliflower, almond meal, egg and flax mixture, garlic powder, onion powder and salt. Process for 30-60 seconds, until well combined.

6. Heat 1 teaspoon of canola oil in a small square cast iron skillet over medium heat. Add half of the cauliflower mixture to the pan, and spread in an even layer with a spatula dipped in water. Repeat with the remaining oil, skillet, and cauliflower mixture.

7. Bake for 12 minutes, until the bread begins to brown on top and is firm to the touch.

Remove from the oven and turn the broiler to low.

8. Grease the tops of the cauliflower bread with nonstick spray. Return to the oven and broil for 3-4 minutes, until golden brown. Let cool in the pans for 10 minutes before topping as desired and serving.

9. Enjoy!

Fiesta Tofu Scramble

Things To Get

for 4 servings

- 1 tablespoon extra virgin olive oil

- 1 red bell pepper, seeded and diced

- 1 jalapeño, seeded and diced

- ¼ medium red onion, diced

- kosher salt, to taste

- 14 oz extra firm tofu(395 g), drained and patted dry

- ½ teaspoon ground turmeric

- 1 teaspoon garlic powder

- ½ teaspoon onion powder

- pepper, to taste

- ¼ cup fresh cilantro leaves(10 g)

- ½ avocado, sliced

- Lime wedge, for garnish

Method

1. Heat the olive oil in a large skillet over medium heat. When the oil is shimmering, add the bell pepper, jalapeño, and red onion.

Season with salt. Sauté for 2 minutes, until the vegetables start to sweat.

2. Crumble the tofu into the pan and stir to break up. Add the turmeric, garlic powder, onion powder, and pepper and stir to combine. Make sure the turmeric evenly coats the tofu to give it an egg-like color.

3. Serve hot with cilantro, sliced avocado, and lime wedges.

4. Enjoy!

High-Protein Sweet And Savory Crepes

Things To Get

for 6 servings

SAVORY RATATOUILLE FILLING

- ½ cup yellow onion(75 g), thinly sliced
- ½ yellow bell pepper, seeded and diced into 1/4 in (6 mm) pieces
- ½ cup roma tomato(100 g), seeded and diced
- ½ cup zucchini(75 g), diced
- ¾ cup japanese eggplant(270 g), about 1 small - diced
- 2 cloves garlic, unpeeled
- 2 tablespoons olive oil
- 2 teaspoons fresh thyme, plus more for garnish
- ½ teaspoon kosher salt, plus more to taste
- ¼ teaspoon freshly ground black pepper, plus more to taste
- ¼ cup goat cheese(55 g), room temperature

SWEET CREPE FILLING

- 1 cup whole milk ricotta cheese(250 g)

- ½ cup strawberry(75 g), finely chopped, plus more for garnish, quartered

- ¼ cup blackberry(35 g), halved, plus more for garnish

- 1 teaspoon lemon zest

- 1 tablespoon honey, plus more for garnish

- whipped cream, for garnish

CREPES

- 6 large eggs

- 1 ½ cups unsweetened coconut milk(360 mL), full-fat canned

- ½ cup coconut flour(60 g)

- 1 tablespoon coconut oil, melted, plus more for greasing

- ½ teaspoon kosher salt

Method

1. If making the savory filling, preheat the oven to 450°F (230°C).

2. In a large bowl, toss together the onion, bell pepper, tomato, zucchini, eggplant, garlic, olive oil, thyme, salt, and pepper. Spread in an even layer on a large baking sheet.

3. Roast the vegetables until they are soft and caramelized, about 18 minutes, flipping halfway through. Set aside to cool.

4. When cool enough to handle, pick the garlic from the vegetables and remove the skin. Add to a large bowl and mash into a paste. Add the goat cheese and stir to combine, then add the vegetables and toss to coat. Season with salt and pepper.

5. Use immediately to fill the crepes, or store in an airtight container in the refrigerator for up to 3 days.

6. If making the sweet filling: In a small bowl, stir together the ricotta, strawberries, blackberries, lemon zest, and honey.

7. Use immediately to fill crepes, or store in an airtight container in the refrigerator up to 3 days.

8. Make the crepes: In a large bowl, combine the eggs, coconut milk, coconut flour, coconut oil, and salt.

9. Using an immersion blender, blend the Things To Get to form a smooth batter, scraping down the sides of the bowl as needed.

10. Preheat a 9-inch (22 cm) nonstick skillet or crepe pan over medium heat. Add just enough

oil to coat the pan, about ½ teaspoon. Swirl the pan to coat evenly.

11. Add ½ cup batter to the hot pan and swirl the pan around again until the batter evenly coats the bottom all the way to the edges. Cook for 4-5 minutes, or until the bottom of the crepe is golden brown in spots and the top is completely cooked through with no raw batter on the surface.

12. Add ¼ cup of your preferred filling to the top left quarter of the crepe. Using a small spatula or spoon, evenly spread the filling over that section, leaving a ½-inch (1 ¼ cm) border along the outside edge.Fold the bottom half of the crepe over the top half, then fold the right (unfilled) side over the left side to form a triangle. Use a rubber spatula to gently transfer

the crepe to a plate. Repeat with the remaining batter and filling.

13. Garnish the savory crepes with more thyme and the sweet crepes with whipped cream, quartered strawberries, blackberries, and honey.

14. Enjoy!

Sweet Potato Breakfast Bars

Things To Get

for 9 servings

- 1 ½ cups mashed sweet potato(375 g)

- 5 tablespoons almond butter

- ⅓ cup maple syrup(110 g)

- ½ teaspoon vanilla extract

- 2 ¼ cups rolled oats(180 g)

- ½ teaspoon cinnamon

- ½ teaspoon ground nutmeg

- ⅓ cup slivered almond(25 g)

- ⅓ cup shredded coconut(35 g)

Method

1. Preheat the oven to 350°F (180°C). Line a 9-inch (23 cm) square baking pan with parchment paper.

2. In a large bowl, stir together the mashed sweet potatoes, almond butter, maple syrup, and vanilla until well combined. Add the oats, cinnamon, and nutmeg and stir until well combined.

3. Transfer the mixture to the baking pan and spread in an even layer with a spatula.

4. Bake for 20 minutes. Remove from oven and top with the slivered almonds and shredded coconut, pressing gently into the bars. Bake for another 10 minutes, until the coconut is lightly toasted.

5. Let cool for 10 minutes, then slice into 9 bars.

6. Enjoy!

Broccoli Cheddar Frittata

Things To Get

for 1 serving

- 2 large eggs

- ⅓ cup broccoli(50 g), finely chopped

- ⅓ cup shredded cheddar cheese(35 g)

- salt, to taste

- pepper, to taste

- ½ teaspoon garlic powder

- chive, sliced, for garnish

Method

1. In a medium bowl, beat the eggs.

2. Add the broccoli, cheddar cheese, salt, pepper, and garlic powder and beat to combine.

3. Heat the mini frying pan over medium heat.

4. Pour the egg mixture into the pan and cover with a small plate.

5. Cook for 10 minutes, or until the egg is set.

6. Transfer to a plate and top with sliced chives.

7. Enjoy!

Chickpea Flour Omelet

Things To Get

for 2 servings

FILLING

- olive oil, for cooking

- ½ cup cremini mushroom(35 g), sliced

- ½ cup cherry tomatoes(100 g), halved

- salt, to taste

- pepper, to taste

- 1 clove garlic, minced

- 2 cups fresh spinach(80 g)

OMELET

- ¾ cup chickpea flour(90 g)

- 1 ½ tablespoons nutritional yeast

- ½ teaspoon baking soda

- ½ teaspoon garlic powder

- ¼ teaspoon turmeric

- ¼ teaspoon salt

- ⅛ teaspoon pepper

- ⅛ teaspoon black salt, kala namak, optional

- 1 teaspoon apple cider vinegar

- ¾ cup unsweetened almond milk(180 mL)

- fresh cilantro, for serving

- salsa, for serving

Method

1. In a medium nonstick saucepan, heat a drizzle of olive oil over medium heat. Once the oil begins to shimmer, add the mushrooms and

tomatoes and cook for 3-4 minutes, until they start to release their juices. Season with salt and pepper.

2. Add a bit more olive oil to the pan, then add the garlic and cook for 2 minutes, until fragrant.

3. Add the spinach and cook for 3-4 minutes, until wilted. Remove the pan from the heat.

4. In a medium bowl, combine the chickpea flour, nutritional yeast, baking soda, garlic powder, turmeric, salt, black salt, apple cider vinegar, and almond milk, and whisk together until mostly smooth.

5. In a medium nonstick saucepan, heat a drizzle of olive oil over medium heat. Once the oil begins to shimmer, add a ½ cup (120 ml) of the omelet batter to the pan. Let cook for 5-7

minutes, or until several bubbles have formed on the surface. Spoon half of the vegetable filling onto one side of the omelet.

6. Using a spatula, fold the omelet in half. Turn off the heat and cover the pan with a lid. Let the omelet steam for 5 minutes, until completely cooked through. Repeat with the remaining omelet batter and filling.

7. Serve the omelets with salsa and fresh cilantro.

8. Enjoy!

Immunity-Boosting Smoothie

Things To Get

for 1 serving

• 4 clementines, peeled

• 1 ripe banana, sliced

• 1 skinny carrot, 6 inch (15 cm), peeled and shaved

• 1 piece fresh ginger, 1 inch (2 cm) peeled and minced

• ¼ cup plain yogurt(60 g)

• 1 tablespoon honey

• salt, to taste

• 1 ½ cups ice(190 g)

Method

1. Add the clementines, banana, carrot, ginger, yogurt, honey, salt, and ice to a blender.

2. Blend until smooth.

3. Serve in a glass or in a bowl topped with fresh fruit.

4. Enjoy!

Lower-Carb Biscuits And Gravy

Things To Get

for 6 servings

BISCUITS

• 2 cups almond flour(190 g)

• 1 tablespoon baking powder

• salt

- ½ cup plain greek yogurt(140 g)

- 2 large eggs

- 2 tablespoons honey

GRAVY

- oil, of choice, for cooking

- 1 lb lean sausage(455 g), or ground turkey

- ¼ cup almond flour(25 g)

- ¼ teaspoon cayenne

- ¼ teaspoon paprika

- ½ tablespoon fresh rosemary, chopped

- ½ tablespoon fresh sage, chopped

- salt, to taste

- pepper, to taste

- 2 cups milk(480 mL), of choice

Method

1. Preheat the oven to 350°F (180°C). Line a baking sheet with parchment paper.

2. Make the biscuits: In a medium bowl, add the almond flour, baking powder, and salt. Whisk to combine.

3. In a separate large bowl, add the Greek yogurt, eggs, and honey. Whisk to combine.

4. Sift the dry Things To Get through a fine-mesh sieve into the wet Things To Get. Mix to combine until fluffy. Do not overmix.

5. Using a large ice cream scoop or a large spoon, scoop dough onto the lined baking sheet, spacing evenly. You should have about 6 biscuits. (If the oven is not ready, keep biscuits in the refrigerator so that they do not spread out and flatten.)

6. Bake for 15-20 minutes, or until golden brown.

7. Make the gravy: Drizzle a bit of oil in a large skillet over medium-high heat, then add the sausage and cook 7-10 minutes, or until browned.

8. Reduce the heat to medium-low and add ¼ cup (25 g) of almond flour, the cayenne, paprika, rosemary, sage, salt, and pepper. Stir to combine, then add the milk.

9. Simmer the gravy until it reaches your desired consistency, stirring occasionally. You can add up to ¼ cup (25 g) more almond flour for a thicker, heartier gravy.

10. Serve the gravy hot, poured over a warm biscuit.

11. Enjoy!

Vegetarian Breakfast Apple Sausages

Things To Get

for 10 links

- 2 tablespoons olive oil, divided

- ½ cup onion(75 g), minced

- 2 cloves garlic, minced

- 1 cup apple(120 g), minced

- 1 cup baby bella mushroom(75 g), minced

- 1 teaspoon fennel seeds

- 1 teaspoon dried rosemary

- 1 teaspoon sage powder

- 1 tablespoon maple syrup

- salt, to taste

* pepper, to taste

* 15 oz cannellini bean(425 g), 1 can, drained and rinsed

* ½ cup chickpeas(100 g), canned, rinsed and drained, or cooked

* 1 cup vital wheat gluten(125 g), or all-purpose flour

Method

1. Heat 1 tablespoon of olive oil in a large skillet over medium heat. Add the onion and garlic and cook for about 4 minutes, until fragrant and the onion is translucent.

2. Add the apples, mushrooms, fennel seeds, rosemary, sage, maple syrup, salt, and pepper and stir to combine. Reduce the heat to medium-low and cook for about 10 minutes, until the mixture is tender and the liquid

released from the mushrooms has evaporated. Remove from the heat and let cool.

3. Add the cannellini beans and chickpeas to a food processor and pulse into a smooth paste.

4. Transfer the bean paste to a large bowl and add the apple/mushroom mixture and vital wheat gluten. Mix with a spatula and then your hands until well combined.

5. Form the sausage mixture into a loaf, wrap in plastic wrap, and refrigerate for 2 hours.

6. Unwrap the chilled sausage mixture and divide into 10-12 equal pieces, depending on what size sausages you would like.

7. Roll a piece between your palms into a sausage shape. Place in the center of a large sheet of plastic wrap and roll the plastic over it so the sausage is completely encased. Twist the

ends of the wrap and knot them together tightly. Repeat for each sausage.

8. Bring a large pot of water to a simmer. Plunge the wrapped sausages in the water and simmer for 45-50 minutes, until the sausages are firm.

9. Remove from the water and let cool for about 5 minutes, then unwrap.

10. Heat the remaining tablespoon of olive oil in a large skillet over medium-low heat. Fry the sausages for 1-2 minutes on each side, until golden brown.

11. Serve immediately or keep wrapped in the refrigerator for up to 4 days.

12. Enjoy!

Cinnamon Apple Quinoa Skillet Bake

Things To Get

for 6 servings

• 2 teaspoons coconut oil, divided

• 2 granny smith apples, diced, plus 1, sliced, divided

• 1 ½ cups quinoa(255 g), uncooked, rinsed well

• ½ cup walnuts(50 g), chopped

• 2 large eggs

• 3 cups unsweetened almond milk(720 g)

• ½ cup applesauce(125 g)

• ⅓ cup maple syrup(110 g)

• 1 teaspoon vanilla extract

• 1 tablespoon cinnamon

- ½ teaspoon ground nutmeg

- 1 pinch salt

Method

1. Preheat the oven to 350°F (180°C).

2. In a large cast-iron skillet, melt 1 teaspoon of coconut oil over medium-low heat. Add the diced apples and let caramelize slightly, stirring occasionally, about 5 minutes. Remove the apples from the skillet and set aside.

3. Melt the remaining teaspoon of coconut oil in the skillet, then add the quinoa and cook until it is well browned and smells toasty, about 10 minutes.

4. Return the apples to the skillet, along with the walnuts. Stir to combine, then remove the skillet from the heat and let cool.

5. In a medium bowl, lightly beat the eggs, then add the almond milk, applesauce, maple syrup, vanilla, cinnamon, nutmeg, and salt. Whisk well to combine.

6. Pour the wet Things To Get into the skillet with the apple quinoa mixture. Arrange the sliced apple on top in a decorative pattern.

7. Bake for 1 hour, until the liquid is absorbed and the quinoa is tender.

8. Remove from the oven and let cool for at least 15 minutes before serving.

9. Nutrition Information, per serving - Calories: 300, Carbs: 45 grams, Dietary fiber: 5 grams, Sodium: 52 mg, Total fat: 10 grams, Total sugar: 21 grams, Total protein: 8 grams

10. Enjoy!

High-Protein Gingerbread Pancakes

Things To Get

for 8 pancakes

- 3 large eggs

- 1 cup cream-style cottage cheese(225 g)

- 1 tablespoon molasses

- 1 tablespoon honey

- 1 teaspoon vanilla extract

- ½ cup oat flour(45 g)

- 1 teaspoon baking powder

- 1 teaspoon ground ginger

- ½ teaspoon ground nutmeg

- ½ teaspoon ground cinnamon

- ¼ teaspoon allspice

- ¼ teaspoon ground cloves

- 1 pinch of kosher salt

- 1 tablespoon chia seeds

- oil of choice, for greasing the skillet

- whipped cream, for serving

- orange segment, for serving

- syrup or sweetener of choice, for serving

Method

1. In a blender, combine the eggs, cottage cheese, molasses, honey, vanilla, oat flour, baking powder, ginger, nutmeg, cinnamon, allspice, cloves, and salt. Blend until well-combined.

2. Pour the batter into a medium bowl and fold in the chia seeds.

3. Heat the oil in a large skillet over medium-high heat. Pour ¼ cup of batter into the pan and cook for 3 minutes, until bubbles start to form and the edges become golden brown. Flip and cook for 3 minutes more, until golden brown on the other side. Repeat with the remaining batter.

4. Top the pancakes with whipped cream, orange segments, and your sweetener of choice.

5. Enjoy!

French Omelette

Things To Get

for 1 serving

- 3 eggs

- salt, to taste

- 1 tablespoon butter, unsalted

- fresh chive, to serve

Method

1. Beat the eggs with the salt until the whites and the yolks are completely combined, with no spots of egg white remaining.

2. Over medium-low heat, melt the butter in a skillet, then pour in the eggs.

3. Using a rubber spatula, constantly scrape the bottom of the pan while shaking the pan in a circular motion to ensure that the eggs cook slowly, forming only small curds, about 1-2 minutes.

4. Once you start to see the bottom of the pan for more than a second after scraping, push the eggs into a round circular shape. Cook until the edges solidify, then tilt the pan and carefully roll the omelette on itself.

5. Invert onto a plate, then sprinkle with chives.

6. Serve immediately.

7. Enjoy!

RECIPES FOR LUNCH ON A CELIAC DIET

Grilled Whole Trout

Things To Get

for 4 servings

- 4 whole trouts, cleaned and gutted

- 2 teaspoons kosher salt

- 1 teaspoon freshly ground black pepper

- 2 lemons, thinly sliced

- 1 bunch scallions, sliced on the bias

- 1 2-inch knob of fresh ginger, peeled and thinly sliced

- ½ bunch fresh cilantro

- 2 tablespoons olive oil, plus more for greasing

SPECIAL EQUIPMENT

- 8 pieces cooking twine, cut into 8-inch (20-cm) lengths

Method

1. On a cutting board, pat the trout dry with paper towels, making sure to get inside the cavity.

2. 2, Generously season the fish with salt and pepper on all sides, including the cavity.

3. Stuff the lemon slices, scallions, ginger, and cilantro in the cavity of each fish.

4. Slip 2 pieces of kitchen twine under each trout and tie to secure the filling inside.

5. Brush both sides of the fish generously with olive oil.

6. Preheat the grill to 350°F (180°C).

7. Dip a paper towel in olive oil and generously rub over the grates of the grill. Place the trout over indirect heat and close the lid. Grill for 6 minutes. Carefully flip the fish over and continue grilling with the lid closed for 6 minutes, until cooked through.

8. Cut the twine off the fish. To remove the bones, take the filling out of the cavity and gently nudge the fish apart. The bones will begin to separate from the flesh. Run your fingers along the bones to loosen, then lift the tail straight up to remove the bones and head, leaving the clean fillets behind.

9. Enjoy!

Chopped Broccoli Salad

Things To Get

for 4 servings

SALAD

- 2 cups small broccoli floret(300 g)

- 1 ½ cups small cauliflower florets(225 g)

- 1 cup brussels sprouts(100 g)

- 1 cup carrot(120 g), chopped

- ½ cup red onion(75 g)

- 4 slices bacon, cooked, roughly chopped (optional)

- ¼ cup shredded sharp cheddar cheese(25 g)

- 3 tablespoons sunflower seeds

- ¼ cup dried cranberries(30 g)

- ¼ cup raw almonds(35 g), sliced

DRESSING

- ½ cup mayonnaise(120 g)

- ¼ cup plain greek yogurt(70 g)

- 2 tablespoons honey

- 2 tablespoons apple cider vinegar

- ½ teaspoon kosher salt

- ½ teaspoon pepper

Method

1. Add the broccoli, cauliflower, Brussels sprouts, carrots, red onion, and bacon, if using, to the bowl of a large food processor. Pulse until the Things To Get are finely chopped, or broken down to your desired consistency. Set aside.

2. Make the dressing: In a medium bowl, stir together the mayonnaise, Greek yogurt, honey, apple cider vinegar, salt, and pepper. Set aside.

3. Add the chopped vegetable mixture to a large bowl, along with the cheddar cheese, sunflower seeds, dried cranberries, and almonds. Drizzle half of the dressing over the salad and toss to combine, adding more dressing as desired.

4. Serve immediately

5. Enjoy!

Pumpkin Ginger Soup

Things To Get

for 4 servings

SOUP

- 1 tablespoon coconut oil

- 1 medium white onion, diced

- 2 teaspoons kosher salt

- 4 cloves garlic, minced

- 1 fresh ginger, 3 in (7 cm) peeled and grated

- 1 jalapeño, seeded and minced

- 2 teaspoons sriracha

- 2 cans unsweetened pumpkin puree

- 2 ½ cups vegetable stock(600 mL)

- 1 can full-fat coconut milk, 13.5 ounce can (380 grams) room temperature

- 1 lime, juiced

- ⅓ cup pepitas(40 g), toasted

CILANTRO COCONUT CREAM

- 1 can coconut cream, 13.5 ounce can (380 grams), chilled

- 1 lime, zested

- 1 cup fresh cilantro leaves(40 g), packed, plus more for garnish

Method

1. In a large pot, melt the coconut oil over medium heat. Add the onion and 1 teaspoon of salt. Cook for 10–15 minutes, until the onions are translucent and softened.

2. Add the garlic, ginger, and jalapeño. Sauté for 3–5 minutes, until fragrant and softened.

3. Add the Sriracha, pumpkin purée, and vegetable stock and stir to combine. Cover the pot, reduce the heat to low, and simmer the soup for 15–20 minutes, until all of the vegetables are completely broken down.

4. While the soup simmers, make the cilantro coconut cream: Add the chilled coconut cream to a liquid measuring cup or tall, narrow container, along with the lime zest and cilantro. Using an immersion blender, blend until the cilantro is completely broken down and the coconut cream turns pale green in color. Chill the cilantro cream in the refrigerator until ready to serve.

5. Remove the soup from heat and stir in the coconut milk. Using an immersion blender, blend the soup until completely smooth. Season with the remaining teaspoon of salt. Stir in the lime juice. Season to taste with more salt, if needed.

6. Ladle the soup into bowls and top each serving with 1 tablespoon of cilantro cream and toasted pepitas.

7. Enjoy!

Salsa-Braised Chicken With Avocado

Things To Get

for 4 servings

• 6 bone-in, skin-on chicken thighs

• kosher salt, to taste

• freshly ground black pepper, to taste

• ½ cup white wine(120 mL)

• 3 cups store bought salsa verde(375 g)

- 2 ripe avocados, pitted, peeled, and cubed

- ¼ cup fresh cilantro(10 g)

- warmed tortilla, for serving (optional)

Method

1. Preheat the oven to 400°F (200°C).

2. Season the chicken thighs all over with salt and pepper. Working in batches if necessary, arrange the thighs skin-side down in a cold, large oven-proof skillet. Place the skillet over medium heat and cook the chicken thighs, undisturbed, until the skin is golden brown and the thighs naturally release from the skillet, 12–15 minutes. Using tongs, transfer the thighs to paper towels.

3. Pour the wine and salsa verde into the skillet and stir to combine with the rendered fat and scrape up any browned bits from the bottom of

the pan, then remove the skillet from the heat. Return the thighs to the skillet, skin-side up, so they are half submerged in the sauce. Transfer the skillet to the oven and bake until the chicken is cooked through and tender and the sauce has reduced and thickened, about 30 minutes.

4. Remove the skillet from the oven, scatter the cubed avocados evenly around the chicken in the sauce, and let the chicken rest in the sauce for 10 minutes.

5. Sprinkle with the cilantro and serve with tortillas on the side, if desired.

6. Enjoy!

Jibarito Sandwich

Things To Get

for 2 sandwiches

STEAK

- 1 orange, juiced

- 1 lime, juiced

- 1 ½ tablespoons olive oil

- 2 ½ teaspoons adobo seasoning

- ½ teaspoon garlic powder

- 3 cloves garlic, minced

- ¼ teaspoon freshly ground black pepper

- 12 oz flank steak(360 g)

- 1 tablespoon vegetable oil

MAYOKETCHUP

- ⅓ cup mayonnaise(80 g)

- ¼ cup ketchup(60 g)

- 2 cloves garlic, minced

- ½ teaspoon garlic powder

- ¼ teaspoon freshly ground black pepper

- ½ teaspoon kosher salt

TOSTONES

- 4 cups vegetable oil(960 mL)

- 2 green plantains, large

- kosher salt, to taste

ASSEMBLY

- 4 slices cheddar cheese, halved lengthwise

- ¼ cup red onion(35 g), thinly sliced

- ½ cup fresh cilantro(20 g)

- ½ cup lettuce(50 g), chopped

- 1 small tomato, thinly sliced

- ¼ avocado, thinly sliced

Method

1. Marinate the steak: In a large bowl, whisk together the orange juice, lime juice, olive oil, adobo seasoning, garlic powder, garlic, and pepper. Add the steak and turn to coat. Cover and refrigerate for 1–2 hours.

2. Make the mayoketchup: In a medium bowl, mix together the mayonnaise, ketchup, garlic, garlic powder, pepper, and salt. Cover and refrigerate until ready to use.

3. Sear the steak: Heat the vegetable oil in a large high-walled skillet over medium-high heat until shimmering.

4. Remove the steak from the marinade and pat dry with a paper towel. Add the steak to the pan and sear for 2-4 minutes on each side until the internal temperature reaches 135°F (55°C). Remove from the pan and set on a cutting board to rest, then slice against the grain into ¼-inch-wide pieces.

5. Make the tostones: Heat the canola oil in a large high-walled skillet over medium heat until it reaches 350°F (180°C).

6. Peel the plantains and cut in half lengthwise. Add the plantains to the hot oil and fry until light golden brown on all sides, 3–4 minutes. Transfer to a paper towel-lined plate to drain.

7. Working 1 at a time, place a plantain half on a cutting board. Place another cutting board on top of the plantain and press down to flatten

until the plantain doubles in width and is about ¼–½ inch thick.

8. Return the oil temperature to 350°F (180°C). Fry the plantains again, 2 at a time, until golden brown and crispy on both sides, 1–2 minutes total. Transfer to a paper towel-lined plate to drain and immediately sprinkle with salt on both sides.

9. Assemble the sandwiches: Spread 1–2 tablespoons of the mayoketchup across a plantain. Top with 2 half-slices of cheddar, and half of the sliced steak, onion, cilantro, lettuce, tomato, and avocado. Spread another 1–2 tablespoons of mayo ketchup on another plantain and top with 2 more half-slices of cheddar. Top the sandwich with the second

plantain. Repeat with remaining Things To Get to make another sandwich.

10. Enjoy!

Gluten-Free Vegan Black Bean Burgers

Things To Get

for 10 servings

• 2 cans black beans, drained, rinsed, and patted dry

• ¼ cup oats(25 g), gluten free if preferred

• ½ cup walnuts(60 g)

• 1 poblano pepper, roughly chopped

• ½ medium onion, roughly chopped

• ½ lime, juiced

- 1 tablespoon onion powder

- 1 tablespoon garlic powder

- 1 teaspoon cumin

- 1 teaspoon fresh parsley

- salt and pepper, to taste

- olive oil, for cooking - optional

Method

1. Preheat the oven to 325 degrees.

2. Spread beans on a lined baking sheet and bake for 15 minutes until slightly dried out. Reserve ½ cup black beans.

3. In a food processor, combine the remaining beans, lime, onion powder, garlic powder, cumin, and parsley. Pulse until mixture comes together. Remove from processor and set aside.

4. In a food processor, combine poblano, onion, oats, and walnuts. Pulse a few times until you reach your desired consistency. I prefer a chunky texture, so I only pulse a couple of times.

5. In a large bowl, combine the bean mixture, oat mixture, the reserved ½ cup black beans, salt, and pepper. Stir until well combined.

6. Using a large cookie or ice cream scoop, scoop the mixture, and form into patties. I used 2 scoops per patty. Place patties on a parchment or waxed paper-lined tray and freeze for one hour.

7. In a non-stick or cast-iron skillet, heat 1 tbsp olive oil over medium heat. Place two frozen patties in a skillet and cook for approximately

4 minutes on each side. Cook remaining burgers, adding a little oil each time.

8. Assemble with desired toppings/bun and serve.

Hummus Caesar Salad

Things To Get

for 2 servings

HUMMUS CAESAR DRESSING

- 4 tablespoons classic hummus

- 1 teaspoon whole grain mustard

- 1 teaspoon minced garlic

- 1.5 teaspoons nutritional yeast

- 1 tablespoon capers, drained and minced

- 1 tablespoon lemon juice

- 1 teaspoon white miso paste, dissolved in 1 1/2 tablespoons hot water

- 2 tablespoons extra virgin olive oil

- kosher salt, to taste

- freshly ground black pepper, to taste

SALAD

- 6 cups mixed greens salad

- lemon juice, to taste

- kosher salt, to taste

- freshly ground black pepper, to taste

Method

1. Make the hummus Caesar dressing: In a medium bowl, combine 4 tablespoons of

hummus, the mustard, garlic, nutritional yeast, capers, lemon juice, miso, and olive oil. Whisk until fully combined. Add another tablespoon of hummus if the dressing is looser than your desired consistency. Season with salt and pepper to taste. The dressing will keep in an airtight container in the refrigerator for up to 1 week.

2. Make the salad: Add the greens to a large serving bowl and lightly season with lemon juice and salt. Generously drizzle the dressing over the salad and toss to coat. Finish with more black pepper, as desired.

3. Enjoy!

Eat Your Feed Fest Pizza

Things To Get

for 8 servings

• A dash of your favorite creators

• 8 ounces viral Tasty classics

• 1 package live cooking demos

• 10 oz local eats(285 g)

• spicy challenge, to taste

Nutrition Info

View Info

Method

1. Tap the "I made this!" button on this recipe.

2. Leave a comment letting us know which Tasty recipe you'd like to enjoy at Eat Your

Feed Fest or why you love Tasty with the hashtag #EatYourFeedFest.

3. Let us know how to contact you using the official entry form (link is located in the tip section).

4. Mark your calendars for November 19 and 20.

5. Keep an eye out for our ticket winner announcement by November 10, 2022.

6. Enjoy live cooking demos hosted by your favorite creators, try some of Tasty's most popular recipes, and eat your way through some of LA's most iconic restaurants and food trucks!

7. Have fun!

Easy Vegan Ramen

Things To Get

for 6 servings

- 1 carton vegetable broth

- 1 carton vegan ramen broth

- 5 cloves garlic, minced

- 1 oyster mushroom, finely chopped

- 4 oz white mushroom(115 g), finely-chopped

- 8 oz clamshell mushrooms(225 g)

- 1 lb gluten-free udon noodles(425 g)

- 3 bunches bok choy, cleaned and cut

- 6 oz fire-roasted corn(175 g)

- 16 oz tofu(450 g), cubed

- 8 oz green onion(225 g), chopped

Method

1. Boil broths together in a large pot.

2. In a sauté pan, add 2 tbsp oil and garlic and cook for 2 minutes or until fragrant. Add minced mushrooms and clamshell mushrooms, cook until soft for about 6 minutes.

3. When broth comes to a boil, add noodles and cook for about 6-8 minutes. Scoop out noodles from pot into a small bowl. Add 1 tbsp of oil and mix noodles to prevent sticking.

4. Add cooked mushroom mix and bok choy, then bring mixture to a boil

5. In a sauté pan, add 1 tbsp of oil and cook corn until roasted and soft.

6. To serve, add noodles and tofu to a bowl, as well as corn. Fill the bowl with broth and top with bok choy and green onions. Serve.

Tteokbokki (Spicy Korean Rice Cakes)

Things To Get

for 4 servings

RICE CAKES (OR USE 1 POUND STORE-BOUGHT RICE CAKES)

- 4 cups sweet rice flour(500 g)

- 1 teaspoon kosher salt

- 1 ½ cups boiling water

- sesame oil, for greasing

TTEOKBOKKI

- 3 cups water(720 mL), plus more for soaking, if needed

- 2 teaspoons dashi powder

- 1 tablespoon gochugaru (Korean red pepper flakes), or to taste

- 1 tablespoon sugar

- 3 tablespoons gochujang (Korean red pepper paste)

- ½ lb fish cakes(225 g)

- 2 eggs hard-boiled eggs

- shredded mozzarella cheese, optional

- 1 green onion, cut into 2-inch (5 cm) pieces

Method

1. Make the rice cakes (alternatively, if using store-bought, jump to step 5): In a medium, microwave-safe bowl, combine the rice flour, salt, and boiling water and mix until well-

combined. Cover the bowl with plastic wrap, leaving an opening for steam to escape.

2. Microwave the dough for 2 minutes. Knead the dough with a spatula, cover again with the plastic wrap, and microwave for another 2 minutes.

3. Grease a flat surface with sesame oil. Pound and knead the dough with a pestle until the dough is smooth and stretchy, about 5 minutes (if you don't have a pestle, you can use another heavy object covered in oiled plastic wrap).

4. Divide the dough into 8 equal portions. Coat the dough in sesame oil, then cover with plastic wrap to prevent them from drying out. Working one at a time, roll each portion into a log, then cut into bite-size pieces and shape each piece as desired. The most common shape

for tteokbokki are cylinders, or you can make fun shapes like hearts. Coat the rice cakes in more sesame oil and spread them out so they don't touch and stick together, then repeat with the remaining dough. You should have about 1 pound. If not using immediately, the rice cakes can be stored in a zip-top freezer bag or wrapped tightly in plastic wrap and frozen for up to three months.

5. Make the tteokbokki: If using frozen rice cakes, soak in room temperature water for 20 minutes.

6. Add the water to a medium skillet and bring to a boil over medium heat. Add the dashi powder and stir until completely dissolved, 1–2 minutes.

7. Add the gochugaru, sugar, gochujang, fish cakes, and rice cakes to the broth. Stir until the gochujang and gochugaru are well-incorporated, then simmer until the broth has reduced to a thick sauce and the rice cakes are soft and squishy, about 5 minutes. During the last 2 minutes of cooking, add the hard-boiled eggs, mozzarella, if using, and green onions. Cover the pan and cook until the cheese is melted.

8. Remove the pan from the heat and serve warm.

9. Enjoy!

Chickpea Sweet Potato Stew

Things To Get

for 4 servings

• 2 tablespoons refined coconut oil

• 1 small onion, diced

• 3 cloves garlic, minced

• 1 teaspoon ginger, minced

• 1 tablespoon sweet paprika

• ½ teaspoon cumin

• ¼ teaspoon dried coriander

• ⅛ teaspoon cayenne

• 15 oz chickpeas(425 g), 1 can, drained and rinsed

• 2 cups sweet potato(400 g), peeled and diced

- 15 oz fire roasted crushed tomato(425 g), 1 can

- 3 cups vegetable broth(720 mL)

- 5 oz fresh spinach(140 g)

Method

1. In large pot or Dutch oven, heat the coconut oil over medium heat. Once the oil begins to shimmer, add the onion and cook for 4-5 minutes, or until the onion is semi-translucent.

2. Add the garlic and ginger, and cook for 2-3 more minutes, until fragrant. Then add the sweet paprika, cumin, coriander, and cayenne and cook for 2 more minutes, until fragrant.

3. Add the chickpeas, sweet potatoes, crushed tomatoes, and vegetable broth, and bring to a boil. Reduce the heat to medium-low and

simmer for 15-20 minutes, or until the sweet potatoes are tender.

4. Add the spinach and stir until wilted.

5. Serve immediately.

6. Enjoy!

Curry Noodle Soup

Things To Get

for 6 servings

• 2 tablespoons refined coconut oil

• 3 cloves garlic, minced

• 1 tablespoon minced fresh ginger

- 2 ½ tablespoons red curry paste

- 15 oz coconut milk(440 mL)

- 3 cups vegetable broth(720 mL)

- 1 tablespoon agave

- 8 oz rice noodles(225 g)

- 7 oz tofu(200 g), cubed

- 2 cups broccoli florets(300 g)

- 1 red bell pepper, thinly sliced

- 1 tablespoon lime juice

- kosher salt, to taste

- chopped fresh cilantro, for garnish

Method

1. In a large pot, melt the coconut oil over medium heat. Once the oil begins to shimmer, add the garlic and ginger and cook for 2-3 minutes, until fragrant.

2. Add the red curry paste and cook for another 2-3 minutes, until aromatic and the garlic and ginger are well-coated.

3. Add the coconut milk and stir well until the curry paste is evenly distributed. Add the vegetable broth and bring to a boil.

4. Once boiling, add the agave and rice noodles and cook for 2 minutes, stirring frequently to prevent the noodles from sticking together.

5. Add the tofu, broccoli, and bell pepper, and stir to combine. Cook for 3-5 more minutes, until the noodles are cooked and the broccoli is tender.

6. Stir in the lime juice and season with salt to taste.

7. Garnish with cilantro and serve immediately.

8. Enjoy!

Bunny-Shaped Apple Slices

Things To Get

for 6 wedges

- 1 apple

- salt water, or lemon water

Method

1. Cut the apple into 6 wedges. Remove the core and seeds.

2. To create the ears: Using a paring knife, make two intersecting slits about ¾ of the way down the skin side of each apple slice. Do not cut too deep.

3. Remove the piece of apple between the slits.
Soak the apple wedges in salt water or lemon
water until ready to eat.

4. Enjoy!

Summer Vegetable Pesto Ribbon Salad

Things To Get

for 4 servings

SALAD

• **2 zucchinis**

• **2 yellow squashes**

• **2 carrots**

• **2 cups grape tomato(400 g)**

• **olive oil, for drizzling**

- salt, to taste

- pepper, to taste

PESTO

- 2 cups fresh basil(80 g)

- 1 cup fresh parsley(35 g)

- ½ cup cashews(65 g)

- 1 clove garlic

- ½ teaspoon salt

- ¼ teaspoon pepper

- 1 tablespoon lemon juice

- ½ cup olive oil(120 mL)

Method

1. Cut the ends off the zucchini. With a vegetable peeler, shave off as many thin slices as possible and transfer a large bowl. Repeat with the yellow squash and carrots.

2. Place the grape tomatoes between 2 large plates or tupperware lids. Press down, securing the tomatoes in place, and use a long, sharp knife to slice the tomatoes in half. Add to the bowl with the shaved vegetables.

3. Drizzle olive oil over the vegetables and season with salt and pepper. Toss to combine.

4. Make the pesto: Add the basil, parsley, cashews, garlic, salt, pepper, lemon juice, and olive oil to a food processor and process until smooth.

5. Spoon the pesto onto the shaved vegetables and mix well with tongs until fully coated and serve.

6. Enjoy!

Thai Tofu Collard Wraps

Things To Get

for 6 servings

WRAPS

- 6 leaves collard green

- 2 tablespoons light soy sauce

- 1 teaspoon garlic powder

- ½ teaspoon red pepper flakes

- 16 oz extra firm tofu(455 g), 1 package, cut into 1/2x2-inch (1x5-cm) strips

- 1 tablespoon sesame oil

- 1 medium cucumber, peeled and julienned

- 1 medium carrot, shredded

- 2 tablespoons fresh thai basil

- 2 tablespoons fresh mint

- 2 scallions, thinly sliced

THAI PEANUT SAUCE

- ½ cup unsweetened natural peanut butter(120 g)

- 1 tablespoon sriracha

- 4 teaspoons toasted sesame oil

- 1 tablespoon honey

- 2 tablespoons lime juice

- 1 tablespoon water

- kosher salt, to taste

Method

1. Bring a large pot of salted water to a boil over high heat.

2. While the water heats up, prepare the collard green leaves. Trim the stems, then, using a paring knife, carefully remove the thick part of the stem from the leaf. Working parallel to the leaf, shave off any excess stem

so that it is flush with the leaf and will roll easily. Repeat with each collard.

3. Blanch each collard green leaf in the boiling water for 1 minute, until softened and bright green. Remove from the water and immediately submerge in an ice bath for 1 minute, or until cool to the touch. Dry the collard greens on paper towels until ready to use.

4. Make the peanut sauce: In a medium bowl, combine the peanut butter, Sriracha, sesame oil, honey, lime juice, water, and salt. Whisk until smooth.

5. In a small bowl, mix together the soy sauce, garlic powder, and red pepper flakes. Pour over the tofu strips and marinate for 15 minutes.

6. Heat the sesame oil in a medium pan over medium-high heat. Add the tofu strips and sear for 2 minutes on each side, until browned. Remove the tofu from the pan.

7. To build the wraps, lay a collard green leaf on a flat surface. Spread 2 teaspoons of peanut sauce across the center of the leaf. Lay 1 strip of tofu on top of the sauce, followed by 3-4 pieces of cucumber, 1 tablespoon shredded carrot, and a bit of mint, Thai basil, and scallions.

8. Fold one side of the leaf over the filling and dollop a bit of peanut sauce on top. Fold the other side of the leaf over the filling, and using the sauce to secure. Fold the bottom of the leaf up and over the filling. Tuck in all of the Things To Get and roll until the bottom half has reached the top of the leaf. Spread a

bit of sauce on the top of the leaf and roll to secure the wrap. Repeat with the remaining Things To Get.

9. Cut in half on the diagonal, then serve with more peanut sauce for dipping, if desired.

10. Enjoy!

Roasted Cauliflower And Curry Soup

Things To Get

for 4 serving

CRISPY CHICKPEAS

• 14 oz chickpeas(395 g), rinsed and drained

• 4 teaspoons curry powder

• 1 teaspoon garlic powder

• 1 teaspoon onion powder

• 1 teaspoon ground coriander

- 1 teaspoon ground turmeric

- 1 teaspoon kosher salt

CURRIED CAULIFLOWER SOUP

- 1 medium head cauliflower, cut into florets

- 1 tablespoon coconut oil, melted, plus 2 tablespoons, divided

- kosher salt, to taste

- freshly ground black pepper, to taste

- 1 small yellow onion, diced

- 1 jalapeño, diced

- 2 cloves garlic, minced

- 3 tablespoons red curry paste

- 14 oz coconut milk(415 mL)

- 4 cups vegetable broth(960 mL)

- sliced scallion, for serving

- chopped fresh cilantro, for serving

• Lime wedge, for serving

Method

1. Make the crispy chickpeas: Preheat the oven to 400°F (200°C).

2. In a medium bowl, toss the chickpeas with the curry powder, garlic powder, onion powder, coriander, turmeric, and salt until well-coated. Transfer the chickpeas to a small baking sheet and spread in an even layer.

3. Roast for 30 minutes, or until the chickpeas are crispy. Remove from the oven and let cool.

4. Make the soup: Increase the oven temperature to 450°F (220°C).

5. Add the cauliflower florets to a medium bowl with the tablespoon of melted coconut oil, salt, and pepper. Toss to coat, then transfer the cauliflower to a baking sheet.

6. Roast for 25 minutes, until browned and tender.

7. Melt the remaining 2 tablespoons of coconut oil in a large pot over medium-high heat. Add the onion and jalapeño and cook until the onion begins to soften, about 2 minutes. Add the garlic and continue to cook for 2 minutes more, until toasted and fragrant.

8. Add the curry paste and cook for 1 minute, stirring to dissolve. Add the coconut milk and vegetable broth and season with salt and pepper. Remove the pot from the heat.

9. Add the roasted cauliflower to a blender, pour in the broth, and carefully purée until smooth.

10. Ladle the soup into bowls. Top with the crispy chickpeas, scallions, and cilantro and serve with lime wedges.

11. Enjoy!

Seared Shrimp And Avocado Salad

Things To Get

for 3 servings

- ½ lb private selection argentine shrimp(230 g), frozen
- 2 tablespoons olive oil
- 1 garlic, minced
- ½ teaspoon kosher salt
- pepper, to taste
- 1 teaspoon lemon zest
- 4 cups mesclun greens(300 g)

- ½ cup quinoa(85 g), cooked

- ½ cup cherry tomato(100 g), halved

- ½ cup avocado(75 g), diced

- ¼ cup chickpeas(50 g), roasted

- 2 tablespoons scallions, sliced, white part only

VINAIGRETTE

- 1 tablespoon shallot

- 2 tablespoons apple cider vinegar

- 1 tablespoon honey

- 2 tablespoons dijon mustard

- kosher salt, to taste

- pepper, to taste

- ½ cup olive oil(120 mL)

Method

1. Add the shrimp to a mesh strainer set in a bowl of cool water and let sit for about 10 minutes to defrost.

2. In a medium bowl, combine the defrosted shrimp, olive oil, garlic, salt, pepper, and lemon zest. Toss until the shrimp are well coated.

3. Heat a medium pan over medium heat. Add the shrimp to the pan and cook for about 1 minute on each side, until pink, opaque, and firm. Remove from the pan and set aside to cool.

4. Make the vinaigrette: In a liquid measuring cup, combine the shallot, vinegar, honey, mustard, salt, and pepper. Whisk until fully incorporated. While whisking, slowly stream in the olive oil until completely emulsified.

5. To assemble the salad, add the mesclun greens to a large bowl. Top with the cooked shrimp, quinoa, cherry tomatoes, avocado, chickpeas, and green onions. Drizzle with the vinaigrette, then toss to combine.

6. Enjoy!

High-Protein Baked Quinoa Bites

Things To Get

for 5 servings

* nonstick cooking spray, for greasing

* 2 cups tuscan kale(200 g)

* 4 cloves garlic

* olive oil, to taste

* ½ teaspoon red pepper flakes

* ⅓ cup sun-dried tomatoes in oil(60 g)

- 4 large eggs

- 4 cups cooked quinoa(680 g), cooled

- 1 cup oat flour(90 g)

- 1 tablespoon dried oregano

- 1 tablespoon dried basil

- 1 tablespoon dried parsley

- 1 tablespoon kosher salt

- ¼ cup freshly grated parmesan cheese(30 g)

Method

1. Preheat the oven to 350°F (180°C). Grease a baking sheet with nonstick spray.

2. Finely chop the kale. Mince the garlic.

3. Heat a drizzle of olive oil in a medium pan over medium heat. Sauté the minced garlic and red pepper flakes for 1 minute, until fragrant. Add the kale and cook until

softened, about 3 minutes. Remove from the heat and set aside.

4. Chop the sun-dried tomatoes and add to the kale mixture.

5. In a large bowl, beat the eggs, then add the quinoa, oat flour, kale mixture, oregano, basil, parsley, salt, and Parmesan cheese. Mix well.

6. Shape the quinoa mixture into 20 small patties. Place on the prepared baking sheet.

7. Bake for 20 minutes, until the patties are golden brown and crispy.

8. Serve as desired. The bites will keep in the fridge for up to 6 days, or in the freezer for up to 1 month.

9. Enjoy!

CELIAC DIET DINNER RECIPES

Low-Carb Eggplant Lasagna

Things To Get

for 12 servings

- 2 large eggplants

- 1 teaspoon sea salt, plus more to taste

- olive oil, to taste

- 5 cloves garlic, minced

- ½ teaspoon red pepper flakes

- 28 oz crushed san marzano tomato(795 g), 2 can

- 6 leaves fresh basil, thinly sliced, plus more for garnish

- 1 large egg

- 15 oz ricotta cheese(425 g), 1 container

- 2 cups shredded mozzarella cheese(200 g), divided

- 1 cup grated parmesan cheese(110 g), divided

- 2 teaspoons italian seasoning

Method

1. Preheat the oven to 375°F (190°C).

2. Cut off the ends of the eggplant, then slice lengthwise about ⅛-inch (3-mm) thick.

3. Sprinkle the eggplant slices with sea salt on both sides and let sit for 10 minutes to draw out moisture. Pat dry with paper towels to remove excess liquid.

4. Lightly grease a griddle pan with olive oil and heat over medium heat. Grill the eggplant

slices for 2-3 minutes on each side, or until grill marks are visible. Remove from the pan and set aside.

5. In a medium saucepan, heat a drizzle of olive oil over medium-low heat, then add the garlic and red pepper flakes. Sauté for about 3 minutes, until the garlic is fragrant but not browned. Add the crushed tomatoes and 1 teaspoon of salt, stirring well to incorporate the garlic and red pepper. Simmer for 10 minutes, reducing the heat if the sauce begins to bubble too much. Add the basil and stir to combine. Remove from the heat and set aside.

6. In a medium bowl, beat the egg, then add the ricotta, 1½ cups (150 g) of mozzarella, ¾ cup (80 g) of Parmesan, and the Italian seasoning. Mix well to combine.

7. Assemble the lasagna. In a 9x13-inch (23x33-cm) baking dish, add enough sauce to cover the bottom of the dish and spread in an even layer. Add a layer of eggplant slices, covering the bottom of the dish completely. It's okay if the eggplant slices overlap slightly. Add a layer of the ricotta mixture and spread in a thin, even layer. Repeat with the remaining Things To Get, finishing with a layer of sauce. Sprinkle the remaining mozzarella and Parmesan on top.

8. Bake for 45 minutes, until cheese is fully melted.

9. Turn the broiler on high and broil for 5 minutes, or until the cheese on top is browned and bubbly.

10. Remove the lasagna from the oven and let rest for 15-20 minutes before serving to give the lasagna time to set.

11. Serve garnished with fresh basil.

12. Enjoy!

Thai Coconut Vegetable Curry

Things To Get

for 8 servings

- 1 tablespoon coconut oil

- 1 red onion, thinly sliced

- 1 medium jalapeno, seeded and finely chopped

- 3 cloves garlic, minced

- 1 orange bell pepper, seeded and cut into thin strips

- 1 large eggplant, ends trimmed, diced

- 3 tablespoons red curry paste

- 1 tablespoon brown sugar

- 13.5 oz light coconut milk(400 mL)

- 28 oz diced tomatoes(790 g)

- 13.5 oz chickpeas(380 g), drained and rinsed

- 5 oz baby spinach(140 g)

- ¼ cup chopped fresh cilantro(10 g)

- cooked brown rice, for serving

Method

1. Melt the coconut oil in a large, high-walled pan over medium heat. Add the onion and cook for 2 minutes, until just beginning to

sweat. Add the jalapeño and garlic, and sauté for 1 minute, until just fragrant. Add the bell pepper and eggplant and cook for 3 minutes, until the eggplant begins to soften.

2. Add the curry paste and brown sugar and stir to coat the vegetables, making sure there are no large clumps of curry paste. Pour in the coconut milk and stir to combine until the milk is stained from the curry paste. Stir in the diced tomatoes and chickpeas and bring to a gentle simmer for 5 minutes.

3. Once the curry is simmering, add the spinach, half at a time, and stir until wilted. Remove the pan from the heat.

4. Garnish the curry with cilantro and serve over brown rice.

5. Nutrition Calories: 212 Total fat: 7 grams Sodium: 368 Total carbs: 34 grams Dietary fiber: 8 grams Sugars: 10 grams Protein: 7 grams

6. Enjoy!

Tofu Turkey

Things To Get

for 6 servings

- 14 oz extra firm tofu(400 g)

- ¾ cup pinto bean(130 g)

- 6 tablespoons nutritional yeast

- ¼ cup soy sauce(60 mL)

- 1 tablespoon poultry seasoning

- 3 cloves garlic, chopped

- ½ teaspoon kosher salt

- 1 teaspoon pepper

- 1 teaspoon onion powder

- 1 cup low sodium vegetable broth(240 mL)

- 2 tablespoons olive oil

- 2 ½ cups vital wheat gluten(310 g)

- ½ cup vegan stuffing(100 g)

- gravy, for serving

SPECIAL EQUIPMENT

- 2 wooden skewers

Method

1. Preheat the oven to 375°F (190°C).

2. Soak the wooden skewers in water to prevent them from burning when baking.

3. Crumble the tofu into a medium bowl lined with a dish towel. Gather the sides of the dish towel and squeeze out as much liquid as possible from the tofu.

4. To a food processor, add the pinto beans, drained tofu, nutritional yeast, soy sauce, poultry seasoning, garlic, salt, pepper, onion powder, and vegetable broth and puree until smooth. With the processor running, pour in the olive oil and continue blending until incorporated.

5. Add the vital wheat gluten to a large bowl, add the mixture from the food processor, and stir until the dough comes together enough that it can be kneaded. Knead for 1-2 minutes,

until most of the cracks have disappeared, then turn out onto a clean surface and shape into a ball. Cut off about ¼ of the dough with a bench scraper and set aside.

6. Transfer the remaining dough to a small glass bowl. Using your hands, form a hole in the center and evenly stretch the edges to help it expand to about 3-4 inches (8 cm) in diameter.

7. Scoop the stuffing into the well, then stretch the sides of the dough over the stuffing to encase completely.

8. Wrap the tofu turkey in parchment paper, then in foil.

9. Divide the reserved dough in half and shape into 2 drumsticks. Insert a wooden skewer in

each one. Wrap the drumsticks in parchment paper, then foil.

10. Set the tofu turkey and drumsticks on a baking sheet and bake for 1 hour, flipping every 20 minutes. Remove the drumsticks after 40 minutes.

11. Serve with gravy.

12. Enjoy!

Winter Vegetable Chili

Things To Get

for 8 servings

• olive oil, to taste

• 1 medium white onion, diced

- kosher salt, to taste

- 3 cloves garlic, minced

- 2 cups parsnip(450 g), peeled and diced

- 3 cups butternut squash(615 g), peeled and diced

- 1 teaspoon paprika

- 2 teaspoons dried oregano

- 2 teaspoons ground cumin

- ¼ teaspoon allspice

- 1 ½ teaspoons chipotle powder

- 28 oz cannellini bean(795 g), drained

- ¼ cup fresh cilantro(10 g), chopped, plus more for garnish

- 4 cups vegetable broth(960 mL)

- shredded cheddar cheese, for garnish

Method

1. In a large, heavy-bottomed pot, heat a drizzle of olive oil over medium heat. Add the onion, season with salt, and cook until the onion starts to sweat and become translucent, 3 minutes. Add the garlic and cook until fragrant, 2 minutes more.

2. Add the parsnips and butternut squash and season with salt, paprika, oregano, cumin, allspice, and chipotle powder. Stir to coat the vegetables with the spices. Cover and cook for 20 minutes, stirring occasionally to prevent sticking, until the vegetables begin to soften.

3. Add the cannellini beans, cilantro, and vegetable broth. Increase the heat to medium-high and bring to a boil for 2 minutes. Reduce the heat to medium-low and simmer for 15

minutes, until the chili is thickened and the vegetables are cooked through.

4. Ladle the chili into bowls and top with cilantro and cheddar cheese.

5. Enjoy!

Vegetarian and Black Bean Quinoa Stuffed Poblanos

Things To Get

for 6 servings

• 6 large poblano chiles

• 1 tablespoon olive oil, plus more for greasing

• ½ medium red onion, diced

- kosher salt, to taste

- 3 cloves garlic, minced

- 2 teaspoons ground cumin

- 1 teaspoon ground coriander

- ½ teaspoon cayenne

- 2 cups cooked quinoa(340 g)

- ¾ cup canned black bean(125 g), drained and rinsed

- ¾ cup fresh corn kernels(130 g)

- ⅔ cup canned tomato sauce(140 g)

- 1 tablespoon lime juice

- ¼ cup coarsely chopped fresh cilantro(10 g), plus whole leaves, for garnish

- ¾ cup shredded monterey jack cheese(75 g)

- sliced avocado, for serving

- Lime wedge, for serving

Method

1. Preheat the oven to 425°F (220°C). Line a baking sheet with a reusable baking mat or parchment paper.

2. Arrange the poblanos on the prepared baking sheet. Roast for 20 minutes, turning occasionally, until the skins begin to turn brown and pull away from the flesh.

3. Meanwhile, make the filling: Heat the olive oil in a large pan over medium heat. Add the red onion, season with salt, and sauté for 3 minutes, until beginning to soften. Add the garlic and sauté for 1 minute, until fragrant. Add the cumin, coriander, and cayenne and stir to coat the vegetables with the spices.

4. Add the quinoa, beans, corn, tomato sauce, and lime juice and season with salt. Stir to combine, then cook until heated through, about 5 minutes. Remove the pan from the heat and stir in the chopped cilantro.

5. Transfer the roasted poblanos to a bowl and cover with a plate or plastic wrap. Steam for 15 minutes.

6. Reduce the oven temperature to 375°F (190°C). Grease a 9 x 13-inch (22 x 33-cm) baking dish with olive oil.

7. Peel the skins off the poblanos. Leaving the stem intact, cut a slit lengthwise down each pepper to form a pouch. With a small spoon, carefully remove the seeds. The poblano flesh will be delicate — it's fine if it tears a bit.

8. Lay the peeled poblanos side by side in the prepared baking dish. Stuff each pepper with about ½ cup of the filling. Top each pepper with 2 tablespoons of Monterey Jack cheese.

9. Bake the stuffed peppers for 15-20 minutes, until the filling is completely warmed through and the cheese is melted and beginning to brown.

10. Garnish the peppers with cilantro leaves and serve with avocado slices and lime wedges alongside.

11. Enjoy!

Homemade Gluten-Free Pasta

Things To Get

for 6 servings

- 3 tablespoons flax meal

- ¼ cup cold water(60 mL), divided plus 9 tablespoons

- 1 cup brown rice flour(125 g), plus more for dusting

- 1 cup quinoa flour(125 g)

- 2 teaspoons xanthan gum

- 1 ½ teaspoons kosher salt, plus more for cooking

- 2 tablespoons olive oil

- sauce of choice, for serving

- grated parmesan cheese, to serve

Method

1. In a small bowl, whisk together the flax meal and 9 tablespoons of cold water. Set aside for 15 minutes, until thickened and gel-like.

2. Meanwhile, in a medium bowl, mix together the brown rice flour, quinoa flour, xanthan gum, and salt. Create a well in the center of the mixture. Pour the flax mixture, remaining ¼ cup (60 ml) cold water, and olive oil into the well. Begin to mix dough together with spatula, then transfer the dough to a clean surface and knead until dough comes together and there are no dry spots remaining. Transfer dough back into bowl and cover. Let rest for 20 minutes to allow the flours and xanthan gum to hydrate.

3. Line a baking sheet with parchment paper.

4. Bring a large pot of water to a rolling boil. Season generously with salt.

5. Divide the dough into 6 equal pieces. Shape each piece into a flat rectangle. Working 1 portion at a time, lightly dust with flour and use a lightly floured rolling pin to roll out to a long, thin rectangle about 3 inches (7 cm) wide and 12 inches (30 cm) long and $\frac{1}{16}$ -inch (1 ½ cm) thick.

6. Feed the rectangle through a pasta roller, starting on the thickest setting and gradually increasing the setting with each pass until the dough is approximately half as thick, but not so thin that it tears.

7. Cut the pasta sheets in half. Feed each half through a fettuccine cutter and twirl each

portion into nests on the prepared baking sheet while you cut the rest of the pasta.

8. Boil the pasta for 2-3 minutes, until al dente but not falling apart.

9. Drain the pasta and toss with the sauce of your choosing.

10. Enjoy!

Golden Chicken Sandwich As Made By Chef Kuniko Yagi

Things To Get

for 2 servings

CHICKEN KARAAGE

- 1 teaspoon fresh ginger, grated

• 1 teaspoon garlic, grated

• ½ teaspoon tamari, or soy sauce

• 2 ½ teaspoons Japanese seasoning salt, divided

• 1 large egg, beaten

• 2 tablespoons potato starch

• 16 oz boneless, skinless chicken thighs(455 g)

• 4 cups rice bran oil(960 mL), for frying

• 2 cups gluten-free flour blend(250 g)

FOR SERVING

• 2 teaspoons red miso

• 2 teaspoons honey

• 2 hot dog buns, halved lengthwise, toasted 7 in (17 cm)

• 12 slices daikon, or pickles of choice

- 10 slices pickled jalapenos

- 2 tablespoons mayonnaise

- ⅔ cup watercress(20 g)

- ½ cup alfalfa sprouts(15 g)

- 2 tablespoons extra virgin olive oil

- 2 tablespoons fresh lemon juice

Method

1. Marinate the chicken: In a medium bowl, whisk together the ginger, garlic, tamari, ½ teaspoon Japanese seasoning salt, egg, and potato starch. Add the chicken thighs and turn to coat. Cover the bowl with plastic wrap and marinate the chicken in the refrigerator for 15 minutes.

2. Fill a medium pot halfway with rice bran oil and heat over medium heat until it reaches 375°F (190°C).

3. Add the gluten-free flour and remaining 2 teaspoons of seasoning salt to a shallow dish and whisk to combine.

4. Coat the marinated chicken thighs in the flour mixture.

5. Fry the chicken thighs, one at a time, in the hot oil for 6–7 minutes, until golden brown and the internal temperature reaches 165°F (75°C). Remove from oil and let drain on a wire rack.

6. In a small bowl, mix together the miso and honey.

7. Spread the miso jam over the bottoms of the toasted hot dog buns. Lay the pickled daikon and jalapeño slices over the miso jam, then

place the chicken karaage on top. Spread the mayonnaise over the top bun and place the watercress on top. Arrange the alfalfa sprouts over the chicken and drizzle with the olive oil and lemon juice.

8. Close the sandwich and secure each side with a wooden skewer. Cut in half, then serve alongside the cole slaw.

9. Enjoy!

Gluten-Free Wild Rice Stuffing

Things To Get

for 10 servings

• 6 tablespoons unsalted butter, divided

- 1 lb Italian sausage(455 g), casings removed and broken up

- 1 medium white onion, diced

- 1 large carrot, diced

- 2 celery stalks, diced

- 1 ½ teaspoons kosher salt, divided

- 3 cloves garlic, mixed

- 1 tablespoon fresh thyme, leaves picked

- 5 leaves fresh sage, minced

- ½ teaspoon freshly ground black pepper

- 1 ¼ cups dried unsweetened cranberry(155 g)

- 1 cup pecan pieces(125 g), toasted

- ½ cup parmesan cheese(55 g)

- 4 cups wild rice medley(920 g), cooked

- 1 ¼ cups chicken stock(300 mL)

- 2 large eggs

- 1 large egg yolk

Method

1. Preheat the oven to 375°F (190°C). Grease a 9 x 13-inch (22.5 x 32.5 cm) baking dish with 1 tablespoon of butter.

2. In a medium pot over medium-high heat, cook the sausage until browned and cooked through, about 8 minutes. Using a slotted spoon, transfer the sausage to a bowl, leaving the rendered fat behind in the pan. Set aside.

3. Lower the heat to medium and melt the remaining 5 tablespoons of butter in the pan with the sausage fat. Once the butter begins to bubble, add the onion, carrot, celery, and ½ teaspoon of salt. Cook for 5–8 minutes, until

the onion is translucent and the carrots begin to soften.

4. Add the garlic, thyme leaves, sage, and black pepper and cook for 2–3 minutes, until the garlic is fragrant. Mix in the dried cranberries, pecans, Parmesan, rice, and sausage and stir well to combine. Remove the pot from the heat.

5. Transfer the stuffing mixture to the prepared baking dish.

6. In a liquid measuring cup, use a fork to whisk together the chicken stock, eggs, egg yolk, and remaining teaspoon of salt.

7. Pour the stock mixture evenly over the stuffing and stir to incorporate. Cover the dish with foil.

8. Bake the stuffing for 40 minutes. Remove the foil and bake for another 10 minutes, until

slightly crispy on top. Remove the stuffing from the oven and let cool for 15–20 minutes before serving.

9. Serve warm.

10. Enjoy!

Zucchini Curry

Things To Get

for 4 servings

- 2 tablespoons oil

- 1 red onion

- 5 cloves garlic

- 2 teaspoons ginger, freshly grated

- 2 teaspoons coriander

- 2 teaspoons smoked paprika

- ½ teaspoon turmeric

- 1 teaspoon cumin

- 3 zucchinis

- 1 can tomato paste, 6 oz (170 g)

- ½ cup vegetable stock(120 mL)

- 1 can full fat coconut milk, 14 oz (395 G)

- salt and pepper, to taste

- fresh cilantro, to garnish, optional

Method

1. First off, dice the onions and garlic and grate the ginger.

2. Then, add oil to a pan over medium heat and when warm, add in the diced onions and saute about 7 -10 minutes, stirring to keep the onions from burning.

3. While the onions are sauteing, dice the zucchini into bite-sized pieces.

4. Then add in the ginger, garlic and zucchini into the pan with the sauteed onions and saute about 5 minutes, stirring often.

5. Add in the coriander, cumin, smoked paprika and turmeric and stir so spices are well incorporated.

6. Then, add in the tomato paste, vegetable stock and coconut milk and stir till all three have combined well. Once it has been mixed well, let this simmer about 3-5 minutes.

7. Season with salt and pepper. If you'd like it a bit spicy, add in a teaspoon of chili powder and mix. Garnish with chopped cilantro and enjoy with roti or naan or rice.

8. Enjoy!

Easy Sweet & Spicy Air Fryer Salmon

Things To Get

for 3 servings

- 3 salmon fillets, 1 in (2.5 cm) thick

- 1 ½ teaspoons coriander

- ½ teaspoon turmeric

- ½ teaspoon chili powder

- 1 tablespoon chili flakes

- ¼ cup honey(85 g)

- ⅛ teaspoon salt and pepper

Method

1. Place honey in a microwave safe dish and heat for 10 seconds until slightly warm.

2. Add in the turmeric, coriander, chili powder, salt, pepper, and chili flakes into the warmed honey and mix very well until all are incorporated.

3. Wash and pat dry the salmon fillets. When salmon fillets are dry, spoon on the honey-chili mixture onto each, making sure to coat the sides as well (this is messy and you will have to wash your air-fryer pan).

4. Then, place the salmon fillets in an air fryer, set temperature to 400°F and set time to 12 minutes. When time is up, remove salmon fillets and enjoy with your favorite sides.

Low-Carb Gluten-Free Cheese Bread Pizza Crust

Things To Get

for 2 servings

• 1 ½ cups shredded mozzarella cheese(170 g), divided

• 2 oz cream cheese(55 g)

• ⅓ cup almond flour(35 g), or coconut flour

• 2 teaspoons baking powder

• ¼ teaspoon garlic powder

• ½ teaspoon italian seasoning

• 1 egg, beaten

TOPPINGS

• ¼ cup tomato sauce(65 g)

• 5 large pepperonis, slices

Method

1. Melt ¾ cup (75 g) mozzarella and cream cheese together in the microwave for 1 minute, stirring every 20 seconds, or until fully melted.

2. Combine almond (or coconut) flour, baking powder, garlic powder, Italian seasoning, and egg. Mix well, then stir in the melted mozzarella until fully incorporated. Shape into a ball, cover, and chill for 30 minutes in the refrigerator.

3. Preheat oven to 425°F (220°C).

4. Place chilled dough on a floured piece of parchment paper. Roll out into a circle about ¼- to ½-inch (6 to 13-mm) thick. Bake for 10 minutes, just until it starts to get golden brown.

5. Top with tomato sauce, remaining mozzarella, and pepperoni, then bake again for

another 5 minutes or until the cheese has melted.

6. Nutrition Calories: 1624 Fat: 142 grams Carbs: 40 grams Fiber: 19 grams Sugars: 10 grams Protein: 59 grams

7. Enjoy!

Dairy-Free Mac 'N' "Cheese"

Things To Get

for 8 servings

DAIRY-FREE "PARMESAN"

• ½ cup raw cashew(65 g)

- ¼ cup nutritional yeast(10 g)

- 1 teaspoon salt

- 1 teaspoon garlic powder

ROASTED GARLIC "CHEESE" SAUCE

- 1 head garlic

- olive oil

- 3 cups cauliflower florets(900 g)

- 2 cups butternut squash(410 g), peeled and chopped into 1-inch (2 cm) cubes

- ½ sweet onion, sliced

- 1 cup carrot(120 g), sliced

- 1 tablespoon lemon juice

- 2 teaspoons dijon mustard

- ¼ cup nutritional yeast(10 g), optional

- 1 teaspoon turmeric

- ½ teaspoon smoked paprika, plus more to taste

- ¼ teaspoon nutmeg

- salt, to taste

- pepper, to taste

- ¼ cup reserved cooking liquid(60 mL)

- ¾ cup almond milk(180 mL)

- 16 oz macaroni(455 g), prepared

Method

1. Preheat the oven to 400°F (200°C).

2. Cut the top edge of 1 head of garlic off, revealing each of the cloves inside the skin.

3. Without removing the skin, place the head of garlic on a foil-lined baking sheet. Drizzle with olive oil. Wrap the garlic up in the foil, making sure it is tightly closed.

4. Bake for 45 minutes, or until the garlic is browned and soft. Set aside to let cool. (When you're ready to add it to the "cheese" sauce, simply squeeze the cloves out of the skin from the uncut end of the bulb, using your fingers.)

5. To make the dairy-free "Parmesan," add the cashews, nutritional yeast, salt, and garlic powder to a food processor or blender. Pulse until you've reached a crumbly, "Parmesan"-like consistency. Set aside.

6. To make the "cheese" sauce, add the cauliflower, butternut squash, onion, and carrots to a large pot of water. Bring to a boil over high heat, then reduce the heat to medium-low, cover and simmer for 15 minutes until the vegetables are tender.

7. Remove the vegetables from the heat and drain, reserving ¼ cup (60 ml) of cooking liquid.

8. To a food processor or blender, add the drained vegetables, roasted garlic cloves, lemon juice, dijon mustard, nutritional yeast, turmeric, smoked paprika, nutmeg, salt, pepper, reserved cooking liquid, and almond milk. Blend until completely smooth, adjusting the seasoning to taste.

9. Pour the sauce over cooked macaroni and stir to combine.

10. Transfer to a large baking dish and sprinkle with "parmesan" and more paprika, if desired.

11. Broil on high for 5-10 minutes, or until the top is golden brown.

12. Enjoy!

Grilled Salmon

Things To Get

for 4 servings

- 8 oz skin-on salmon(225 g), 4 fillets

- fine sea salt

- freshly ground black pepper

- 2 lemons, halved crosswise

Method

1. Heat a grill to medium-high heat.

2. Season the salmon with salt and pepper.

3. Brush the grill grates with oil and place the salmon, skin side down on the oiled grates.

4. Grill until lightly browned, 3-5 minutes, then gently flip and continue to cook until just opaque in center.

5. Add the lemon halves to the grill, cut side down and grill until lightly charred, about 2 minutes.

6. Enjoy!

Gluten-Free Grilled Flatbread Pizzas

Things To Get

for 8 servings

- 1 ½ cups warm water(360 mL)

- 1 packet active dry yeast

- 2 large large egg

- 2 tablespoons olive oil

- 3 ¼ cups gluten-free flour blend(405 g)

- topping of your choice

Method

1. Pour the water into a large bowl and add the yeast. Let sit for 2 minutes while the yeast activates. The mixture should become foamy and some of the yeast will sink in the water.

2. Add the eggs and oil. Whisk until smooth.

3. Add the gluten-free pizza dough mix and stir with a wooden spoon until well-combined.

4. Use a bowl scraper to divide the dough in half. Grease 2 medium bowls with olive oil.

Place each dough half in a bowl and top with another drizzle of oil.

5. Toss the dough to evenly coat in oil, then cover the bowls with clean kitchen towels. Let rise for 20 minutes, until the dough has expanded, but not quite doubled in size.

6. Heat a grill pan over high heat.

7. Turn a dough portion onto a lightly floured pizza peel or other flat surface, like a cutting board or cookie sheet. Dust the dough with more flour and roll out into a 10-inch (25-cm) round, or whatever size will fit the pan you're working with.

8. Carefully slide the dough onto the grill pan. Grill each side for 6-8 minutes, until dark grill marks form. Remove from the heat. Repeat with the remaining dough.

9. Top with your desired toppings, slice, and serve.

10. Enjoy!

Vegetarian Gumbo

Things To Get

for 5 servings

• 6 tablespoons olive oil, divided

• 1 cup yellow onion(150 g), diced and divided

• 10 oz cremini mushroom(280 g), finely chopped

• 6 cloves garlic, minced and divided

• 2 tablespoons low sodium soy sauce

- 2 teaspoons dried thyme, divided

- 2 teaspoons smoked paprika, divided

- 1 teaspoon dried oregano, divided

- ½ teaspoon cayenne pepper, divided

- 3 teaspoons vegan worcestershire sauce, divided

- 1 teaspoon liquid smoke, divided

- ½ teaspoon salt, plus more to taste, divided

- ¾ teaspoon pepper, divided

- 15 oz cannellini bean(425 g), 1 can, drained and rinsed

- ¾ cup bread crumbs(85 g)

- ⅓ cup vital wheat gluten(40 g), or bread crumbs

- 3 ½ cups vegetable broth(840 mL), plus 2 tablespoons, divided

• 3 tablespoons all purpose flour

• 1 stalk celery, diced

• 2 cups okra(200 g), sliced into 1/2-in (1 cm) rounds

• 1 green bell pepper, seeded and diced

• 1 ½ cups tomato(300 g), crushed

• 15 oz red kidney bean(425 g), 1 can, drained and rinsed

• brown rice, cooked, for serving

• fresh parsley, chopped, for serving

Method

1. In a large pot, heat 1 tablespoon of olive oil over medium heat. Once the oil begins to shimmer, add ½ cup (75g) diced onion and cook for 3-4 minutes, until semi-translucent.

2. Add the mushrooms and cook for 5 minutes, until most of the juices have evaporated.

3. Add 2 cloves of minced garlic, the soy sauce, 1 teaspoon thyme, 1 teaspoon paprika, ½ teaspoon oregano, ¼ teaspoon cayenne, 2 teaspoons vegan Worcestershire sauce, ½ teaspoon liquid smoke, ½ teaspoon salt, and ¼ teaspoon pepper and cook for another 4-5 minutes, until all of the liquid has evaporated and the spices are fragrant.

4. Add the cannellini beans to a medium bowl and mash until mostly smooth (a few lumps are okay). Then, add the mushroom mixture, bread crumbs, vital wheat gluten, and 2 tablespoons vegetable broth and mix well until combined. Use your hands to knead the mixture until cohesive, then begin to roll about

a tablespoon at a time of the mixture into "meatballs".

5. In the same large pot, heat 3 tablespoons of olive oil over medium heat. Once the oil begins to shimmer, add the meatballs and cook for about 5 minutes on each side, until golden brown. Remove the meatballs from the pot and set aside.

6. Add the remaining 2 tablespoons of olive oil to the pot, along with the flour. Stir the roux continuously with a wooden spoon for about 3-4 minutes, until the consistency resembles wet sand.

7. Add the remaining ½ cup (75g) diced onion, the celery, and the okra to the pot and cook for 4-5 minutes, until the onion is semi-translucent.

8. Add the remaining 4 cloves of minced garlic and the green bell pepper and cook for another 3-4 minutes, until the garlic is fragrant.

9. Add the remaining teaspoon of vegan Worcestershire sauce, ½ teaspoon liquid smoke, 1 teaspoon thyme, ½ teaspoon oregano, 1 teaspoon paprika, ¼ teaspoon cayenne, and ½ teaspoon pepper and cook for 4 more minutes, until the spices are fragrant.

10. Add the crushed tomatoes and stir until combined. Then, add the red beans and add the remaining 3½ cups (840ml) vegetable broth and stir until well combined. Simmer on low heat for 30 minutes, stirring from time to time, until the gumbo has thickened.

11. Season with salt to taste. Then, add the meatballs and stir to incorporate.

12. Serve over rice and garnish with parsley.

13. Enjoy!

Pesto And Prosciutto Zucchini Linguine

Things To Get

for 2 servings

• 2 medium zucchinis, washed and trimmed

• 2 cups spinach(80 g)

• 1 cup fresh basil leaves(40 g), plus more for garnish

• ½ cup pine nuts(60 g)

• ¼ cup shredded parmesan cheese(25 g), plus more for garnish

• 2 cloves garlic, minced

- ¼ cup olive oil(60 mL), plus more as needed

- 2 tablespoons lemon juice

- salt, to taste

- pepper, to taste

- 1 cup cherry tomatoes(200 g), halved

- 2 slices prosciutto, torn or cut into bite-size chuncks

- lemon wedge, for garnish

Method

1. Use a spiralizer to cut the zucchini into zoodles. Add the zoodles to a serving bowl and set aside.

2. Make the pesto: in a food processor or blender, add the spinach, basil, pine nuts, Parmesan, garlic, olive oil, lemon juice, salt,

and pepper. Blend to desired consistency, adding more olive oil as needed.

3. Scoop the pesto over the zucchini noodles, then add the cherry tomatoes and prosciutto. Toss until the zoodles are well-coated.

4. Sprinkle with Parmesan and garnish with basil and lemon wedges.

5. Enjoy!

Eggplant Potato Tomato Stew

Things To Get

for 5 servings

- 4 medium yukon potatoes

- 2 medium eggplants, chopped

* 2 red bell peppers, seeded and chopped

* 5 tablespoons olive oil, divided

* 1 teaspoon salt, plus more to taste, divided

* ¾ teaspoon pepper, plus more to taste, divided

* 1 medium yellow onion, diced

* 1 tablespoon tomato paste

* 3 cloves garlic, minced

* 1 teaspoon smoked paprika

* 15 oz chickpeas(425 g), 1 can, drained and rinsed

* 3 medium beefsteak tomatoes, diced

* 1 ½ cups low sodium vegetable broth(360 mL)

* fresh parsley, for serving

Method

1. Preheat the oven to 400°F (200°C).

2. With a sharp knife, score a ring around each potato, just deep enough to break the skin. Place the potatoes in a medium pot of cold water. Bring to a boil and cook for about 8 minutes, until about halfway cooked.

3. Drain the potatoes, and rinse with cold water. Peel off the skin.

4. Cut the potatoes into ½-inch (1 cm) pieces and set aside.

5. Divide the eggplant and bell peppers between 2 baking sheets and spread in an even layer. Drizzle with 4 tablespoons of olive oil, and season with salt and pepper to taste. Toss with your hands to coat.

6. Bake for 25 minutes, flipping halfway through.

7. Heat the remaining tablespoon of olive oil in a large pot over medium heat. Once the oil begins to shimmer, add the onion and cook for 3-4 minutes, until semi-translucent.

8. Add the tomato paste and stir until well distributed, then add the garlic, paprika, 1 teaspoon salt, and ¾ teaspoon pepper, and cook for another 2-3 minutes, until fragrant.

9. Add the potatoes, chickpeas, and tomatoes, and stir to incorporate.

10. Stir in the vegetable broth and cover. Reduce the heat to low and cook for 20 minutes, until the potatoes are tender.

11. Add the roasted eggplant and bell pepper, and stir to combine. Cook for another 5-10 minutes, until the tomatoes have mostly broken down.

12. Ladle into bowls, garnish with parsley, and serve. Or, transfer the stew to resealable containers and store in the fridge for up to 5 days or freezer for up to 3 months.

13. Enjoy!

Keto-Friendly Lasagna Dome

Things To Get

for 8 servings

- 3 tablespoons olive oil

- 1 cup carrot(110 g), grated

- 1 medium yellow onion, diced

- 2 lb ground beef(910 g)

- 1 ½ teaspoons dried oregano

- ½ teaspoon red pepper flakes

- black pepper, to taste

- 4 cloves garlic, minced

- ½ cup dry red wine(120 mL)

- 28 oz crushed tomato(795 g), 1 can

- ½ cup fresh basil(20 g), chopped

- salt, to taste

- 1 large head savoy cabbage, eaves separated and stems trimmed

- 1 egg, beaten

- 2 cups whole milk ricotta cheese(500 g)

Method

1. Preheat the oven to 375°F (190°C).

2. Heat the olive oil in a large pan over medium heat. Add the carrot and onion, and cook until

the vegetables have softened slightly, 8-10 minutes.

3. Add the beef and season with the oregano, red pepper flakes, and pepper. Use a wooden spoon to break the beef into smaller pieces, and cook until browned, about 10 minutes.

4. Add the garlic and cook until fragrant, 2-3 minutes.

5. Deglaze the pan with red wine, scraping up any browned bits from the bottom of pan.

6. Once the wine has reduced by half, stir in the crushed tomatoes. Cook until sauce has thickened, stirring frequently, about 10 minutes.

7. Stir in the basil, then remove the sauce from the heat and let cool.

8. Bring a large pot of salted water to a boil. Working in batches, add the cabbage leaves, using tongs to submerge them in the water. Cook until the leaves have softened and are flexible, 1-2 minutes. Drain well and pat dry with a paper towels.

9. Stir the egg into the cooled meat sauce.

10. Place the largest cabbage leaf on the bottom of a 9-inch (23-cm) round baking dish. Line the exposed sides and bottom of the pan with more cabbage leaves.

11. Spoon in ¼ of the meat sauce, spreading evenly. Dollop ¼ of the ricotta on top of the sauce. Cover with cabbage leaves. Repeat with the remaining sauce, ricotta, and cabbage to make 3 more layers.

12. Fold any overhanging cabbage leaves toward the center of the pan.

13. Bake on the middle rack of the oven for 1 hour, until lightly browned on top. Let cool for 20 minutes.

14. To serve, place a serving plate over the baking dish and invert the chou farci onto the plate. Remove the pan, then slice into wedges and serve.

15. Enjoy!

DESSERTS RECIPES SUITABLE FOR A CELIAC DIET

Nian Gao

Things To Get

for 1 7-inch round cake

• 2 tablespoons vegetable oil, divided, plus more for frying (optional)

• 3 cups water(720 mL), divided, plus more as needed

• 2 slices peeled fresh ginger

• 12.5 oz brown rock sugar(360 g), or 2 cups (packed) dark brown sugar

• 1 lb glutinous rice flour(425 g)

• 1 dried jujube

• roasted sesame seed, for garnish

Method

1. Grease a 7-inch round, nonstick baking dish with 1 tablespoon of the oil.

2. In a medium saucepan, combine 2½ cups (500 ml) of water and the ginger and bring to a boil over high heat. Reduce the heat to medium, cover, and simmer for 10 minutes.

3. Uncover the pot, add the rock sugar, and continue simmering until the sugar melts completely, stirring occasionally (if using rock sugar bricks, break the bricks into smaller pieces with your hands to allow it to melt more quickly).

4. Remove the pot from heat and discard the ginger. Stir in the remaining ½ cup of water to help the syrup cool down, then let sit until the

temperature reaches 120°F (50°C), about 10 minutes.

5. While the syrup is cooling, prepare a steamer by filling the bottom with water (make sure there is enough to steam the cake for about 1 hour, but not so much that it touches the bottom of the pan) and bringing the water to a boil over medium heat. Alternatively, you can use a rice cooker to steam the nian gao (see instructions below).

6. Add the glutinous rice flour to a large bowl and drizzle in the remaining tablespoon of vegetable oil. Mix the oil in with your hands.

7. Once the syrup has cooled, gradually add it to the flour mixture, mixing with your hands or a rubber spatula to combine as you go. Once all of the syrup has been added, continue

mixing until the batter is well-combined and no lumps remain. It should be thin enough to drizzle; if needed, stir in additional water, ¼ cup at a time. Pour the batter through a mesh strainer into a separate large bowl to remove any remaining clumps of flour.

8. Pour the batter into the prepared baking dish and tap on the countertop to release any air bubbles. If needed, puncture any air bubbles on the surface with a chopstick. Cover the pan with aluminum foil, if desired (this will prevent any condensation from dripping onto the cake).

9. Place the nian gao in the steamer, cover, and steam for 45–60 minutes, adding more water to the steamer as needed, until the cake is light brown and sticky when a wooden skewer is

inserted into the center, but holds its shape. The cake may puff up, but will settle once cooled. Carefully remove the pan from the steamer and let the cake cool for about 20 minutes.

10. If desired, invert the pan onto a plate to remove the cake (or serve directly from the pan). Place the jujube at the center of the cake and sprinkle with sesame seeds. Slice and serve fresh for a sweet, sticky, and chewy texture. Alternatively, if left covered at room temperature for a day, the cake will become firmer. Slice and pan-fry the pieces in a bit of neutral oil for a crispy and chewy treat.

11. Leftover cake will keep covered at room temperature for up to 3 days, or in an airtight container the refrigerator for up to 1 week.

12. Rice cooker instructions: Pour the batter into a pan that will fit inside the basin of the rice cooker (make sure it is deep enough to hold all of the batter). Set a ceramic ramekin or stacked mason jar lids in th bottom of the rice cooker, place the pan on top, then pour water into the base of the rice cooker until it reaches just below the nian gao pan. Close the lid and cook the cake on the white rice setting.

13. Enjoy!

Low Fat, Gluten-Free Vegan Apple Cider Donuts

Things To Get

for 6 servings

DRY:

- 1 ½ cups millet flour(185 g)

- 2 teaspoons baking powder

- 1 teaspoon ground cinnamon

WET

- ½ cup apple cider(120 g)

- 5 oz vanilla soy, or almond yogurt

- ½ teaspoon vanilla extract

- ⅛ teaspoon liquid Stevia

COATING (OPTIONAL)

- ½ cup maple sugar(165 g)

- 1 teaspoon ground cinnamon

Method

1. Pre-heat the oven to 350 degrees F.

2. Sift the dry Things To Get, then stir in a medium bowl.

3. In a small bowl, combine the wet Things To Get, and stir well. Then, add the wet to the dry Things To Get and mix until combined.

4. Pour the batter evenly into a six-donut baking pan.

5. Bake for 10-15 minutes, until firm on top and edges. Once baked, remove from the oven.

6. While the donuts are resting, combine the maple sugar and cinnamon in a small bowl and coat the warm donuts on both sides in the coating.

7. Serve.

Homemade Date Donuts

Things To Get

for 6 servings

• 10 mejdool dates, pitted

• ¼ cup tap water(60 mL)

• ⅓ cup peanut butter(80 g), or nut butter of choice

• 4 tablespoons cocoa powder

• 2 tablespoons flaxseed meal

• ½ teaspoon baking soda

• 1 pinch salt

• topping of your choice, Chocolate/Vegan Chocolate melted in the microwave OR equal parts of Cocoa Powder & Coconut Oil

Method

1. Preheat the oven to 180°C

2. Add the pitted dates, tap water and lemon juice to a food processor or blender. Blitz until a paste forms. You may have to stop to scrape down the edges in between.

3. Add the peanut butter, cocoa powder, flaxseed meal, baking soda and salt. Blitz again until well combined

4. Grease a donut tray or mini cupcake tray with cooking spray. Use a spoon or wet hands to split the dough equally

5. Bake for 15 minutes, then let the donuts sit in a turned off oven for 5 minutes.

6. Let cool, then remove from the tray and top with melted chocolate or a mix of melted coconut oil & cocoa powder

Vegan Rose White Chocolate Chip Oats Cookies

Things To Get

for 24 cookies

- 2 cups gluten-free oat flour(250 g)

- ½ teaspoon baking soda

- ½ teaspoon baking powder

- ¼ teaspoon salt

- ¼ cup melted coconut oil(60 mL)

- 1 tablespoon rose water

- ¼ cup coconut sugar(50 g)

- ¼ cup pure maple syrup(85 g)

- 2 flax-eggs, (2 tablespoons ground flax + 6 tbsp water, whisked together, set for 15 minutes)

- 2 tablespoons dried rose petal

- 1 ½ cups vegan white chocolate chips(215 g)

Method

1. Preheat the oven to 350°F. Line a baking sheet with parchment paper and set it aside.

2. Whisk together all of the dry Things To Get in a mixing bowl: oat flour, baking soda, baking powder, and salt.

3. In a separate, large mixing bowl, combine the wet Things To Get: coconut oil, coconut sugar, maple syrup, flax eggs, and rose water and mix until thoroughly combined.

4. Combine the dry and wet Things To Get in a mixing bowl. Whisk until everything is well mixed. Stir in the chocolate chips and rose petals.

5. Cover the cookie dough bowl. Allow to remain at room temperature for 10 minutes to allow the dry mixture to absorb the liquid mixture.

6. Scoop about 2 teaspoons of cookie dough onto the baking sheet lined with parchment paper. Use your palm to softly flatten the cookies into a circular disc, they will not spread while baking. Chocolate chips can be pressed into the tops of the cookies if desired.

7. Bake for 8-10 minutes, or until lightly golden brown and set. With a flat, heatproof spatula, remove the cookies from the baking sheet and set them on a cooling rack to cool. Allow to thoroughly cool and serve.

Easy Slow Cooker Chili Cheese Fries

Things To Get

for 6 servings

SLOW COOKER CHILI

• 1 lb cooked lean ground beef(455 g), or turkey

• 1 cup yellow onion(150 g), diced

• 2 cans diced tomato, with green chiles

• 1 can kidney bean, drained and rinsed

• 1 can black beans, drained and rinsed

• 2 tablespoons chili powder

• 2 teaspoons ground cumin

• 2 teaspoons kosher salt

QUICK PICKLED JALAPEÑOS

- ½ cup water(120 mL)

- ½ cup distilled white vinegar(120 mL)

- 1 tablespoon kosher salt

- 1 tablespoon sugar

- 2 cloves garlic

- 2 strips lime zest

- 6 jalapeñoes, sliced into 1/2 in (1 1/4 cm) round

CHILI CHEESE FRIES

- 1 bag frozen french fries, preferably crinkle cut

- 1 cup shredded mexican cheese blend(100 g)

- ½ cup sour cream(120 g)

- 4 scallions, thinly sliced

SPECIAL EQUIPMENT

- slow cooker

Method

1. Make the chili: In a slow cooker, combine the ground beef, onion, diced tomatoes, kidney beans, black beans, chili powder, cumin, and salt. Cover and cook on low, stirring often, for about 6 hours, or until the onions are tender.

2. While the chili cooks, make the quick pickled jalapeños: In a small saucepan, combine the vinegar, water, salt, sugar, garlic, and lime zest. Bring the mixture to a boil over medium-high heat, then reduce the heat to low and simmer until the salt and sugar have dissolved, about 2 minutes.

3. Add the jalapeños to a medium heatproof bowl or large mason jar. Carefully pour the pickling liquid over the jalapeños, making sure

they are fully submerged. Let the pickles cool to room temperature, about 1 hour. Cover the bowl with plastic wrap or seal the jar and transfer to the refrigerator until ready to use. The pickled jalapeños will keep in the refrigerator for up to 2 weeks.

4. Make the chili cheese fries: Preheat the oven according to the French fry package instructions.

5. Spread the French fries in an even layer on a rimmed baking sheet. Bake for 3 minutes less than the package instructs.

6. Remove the fries from the oven and top with several large scoops of chili. Sprinkle the shredded cheese evenly over the top. Return to the oven for about 5 minutes, or until the cheese has melted completely.

7. Dollop the sour cream on top of the chili cheese fries, then garnish with the scallions and pickled jalapeños. Let cool slightly, then serve directly off of the pan.

8. Enjoy!

Chicken Tinga Sheet Pan Quesadilla

Things To Get

for 12 servings

- 2 tablespoons olive oil

- 1 medium white onion, diced

- 2 cloves garlic, minced

- 4 cups shredded rotisserie chicken(500 g)

- 1 jar Pace® Picante Sauce, divided

- 1 tablespoon adobo sauce, to taste

- ¼ teaspoon kosher salt

- nonstick cooking spray, for greasing

- 12 flour tortillas, 9 in (22 cm)

- 2 cups refried beans(280 g), optional

- 3 cups shredded mexican cheese blend(300 g)

- ⅓ cup melted unsalted butter(75 g)

- 1 cup Pace® Chunky Salsa(336 g), for topping

- ½ cup sour cream(120 g), or crema, for topping

- ¼ cup fresh cilantro(10 g), for topping

Method

1. Preheat the oven to 425°F (220°C). Line a baking sheet with foil and grease with nonstick spray.

2. Make the chicken tinga: Heat the olive oil in a large skillet over medium heat. Add the onion and garlic and sauté for 4 minutes, or until the onion is translucent and starting to brown. Add the shredded chicken, 1¾ cups (415 G) Pace® Medium Picante Sauce, the adobo sauce, and salt, and stir to combine. Bring to a simmer and cook for 5 minutes, stirring often, until the chicken is heated through. Remove the pan from the heat.

3. Assemble the quesadilla: Place 8 tortillas around the edges of the prepared baking sheet so about half of each tortilla hangs over the side of the pan. Place another 2 tortillas in the center to cover the pan completely.

4. Spread the refried beans on top of the tortillas inside the baking sheet, making sure to

spread all the way to the corners. Sprinkle 1½ cups Mexican cheese over the beans and drizzle with the remaining cup of Pace® Medium Picante Sauce. Spread the chicken tinga evenly on top, then cover with the remaining 1½ cups Mexican cheese.

5. Place the remaining 2 tortillas, over the filling at the center of the baking sheet, overlapping slightly. Carefully fold the overhanging tortillas around sides of the pan over the center tortillas to cover the filling completely, tucking in the corners.

6. Brush the top of the tortillas with the melted butter, then place another baking sheet over the tortillas to keep in place.

7. Bake for 20 minutes, then remove the top baking sheet and bake for another 15 minutes,

or until the tortillas are browned. Remove from the oven and let rest in the pan for 10 minutes.

8. Use the foil to lift the quesadilla onto a cutting board, then remove the foil.

9. Drizzle the quesadilla with the Pace® Chunky Salsa and sour cream, then top with the cilantro. Slice into 12 rectangles and serve.

10. Enjoy!

Sweet And Sour Chicken Lettuce Cups

Things To Get

for 4 servings

• 2 boneless, skinless chicken breasts

• 2 teaspoons salt, plus more to taste

• 2 teaspoons black peppercorn

• ½ medium sweet onion, halved

• ½ medium sweet onion, diced

• 6 cloves garlic, divided, 4 whole and 2 minced

• 2 bay leaves

• 6 cups water(1.4 L)

• 1 tablespoon oil

• ¼ cup low sodium soy sauce(60 mL)

• ¼ cup honey(85 mL)

• ½ cup lime juice(80 mL)

• 4 large leaves romaine lettuce, for serving

• ¼ cup scallion(25 g), sliced

Method

1. Place the chicken breasts, salt, peppercorns, halved onion, whole garlic cloves, bay leaves, and water in a large pot.

2. Cover the pot and bring to a simmer over medium heat.

3. Once the water is simmering, cook for 10 minutes, until the chicken registers 165°F (74°C) when pierced with an instant-read thermometer.

4. Transfer the chicken to a cutting board and discard the cooking liquid. Using 2 forks, pull the chicken apart until shredded.

5. In a large nonstick pan, heat the oil over medium-high heat until shimmering.

6. Add the diced onion and a pinch of salt and sauté until softened, about 2 minutes.

7. Add the minced garlic and sauté until fragrant, about 30 seconds.

8. Add the soy sauce, honey, and lime juice and stir until the mixture has thickened slightly, about 2 minutes.

9. Add the shredded chicken and mix until everything is well incorporated.

10. Remove the pan from the heat and let the chicken cool for 5 minutes before spooning into the lettuce leaves.

11. Top with sliced scallions.

12. Enjoy!

Easy Shrimp Ceviche

Things To Get

for 2 cups

• 10 limes

• 1 lb shrimp(455 g), peeled, deveined, and diced

• 2 teaspoons kosher salt

• 2 jalapeñoes, seeded and minced

• 1 small red onion, diced

• 2 cups cherry tomato(400 g), chopped

• fresh cilantro leaf, for garnish, optional

• tortilla chip, for serving

Method

1. Halve the limes, then juice using a citrus press or a pair of kitchen tongs. You should have about 1 cup (240 ML) total.

2. In a medium bowl, combine the shrimp, lime juice, salt, jalapeños, onion, and tomatoes. Mix well.

3. Cover and refrigerate for about 4 hours, until the shrimp is opaque and firm.

4. Serve the ceviche chilled. Garnish with cilantro, if desired, and serve with tortilla chips.

5. Enjoy!

Slow Cooker Cheesy Chicken And Bean Dip

Things To Get

for 4 servings

- 1 rotisserie chicken, shredded

- 2 cups refried beans(475 g)

- 1 cup cream cheese(225 g)

- 1 cup sour cream(230 g)

- 2 cups shredded cheddar cheese(200 g)

- 1 tablespoon taco seasoning

- tortilla chip

Method

1. Set aside 1 cup (100 grams) of shredded cheddar cheese. Combine all other Things To Get in crockpot and mix well.

2. Cook on high for 1 ½ hours. Stir dip and add remaining cheddar cheese on top. Let cheese melt then eat with tortilla chips

3. Enjoy!

Thai Street Wings As Made By Chef Arnold Myint

Things To Get

for 4 servings

- 3 lb chicken wings(1.3 g), wings and drumettes separated

- ¼ cup fish sauce(60 mL)

- ¼ cup low sodium soy sauce(60 mL)

- ¼ cup dark soy sauce(60 mL)

- ½ cup palm sugar(100 g)

- 2 stalks lemongrass, split in half and cracked to release aromatics

- ½ cup fresh cilantro leaves(20 g), torn

• 1 teaspoon freshly ground black pepper

• 20 cloves garlic, peeled and smashed

• thai chili-lime sauce, store bought

• sticky rice, and assorted crunchy vegetables, for serving

Method

1. Add the chicken wings, lemongrass, cilantro, garlic, pepper, soy sauce, fish sauce, low-sodium soy sauce, and palm sugar to a large zip-top bag. Seal the bag and massage the chicken to coat. Marinate in the refrigerator for at least 2 hours, up to overnight.

2. Preheat the oven to 350°F (180°C). Place your oven rack on the upper third of the oven and place a metal cooling rack inside a rimmed baking sheet.

3. Arrange the marinated chicken wings on the rack. Transfer to the oven and bake for 15 minutes, until browned and the internal temperature reaches 165°F (75°C). Turn the oven to broil and broil the wings until the skin starts to char slightly, about 2 minutes. Transfer to a platter and serve immediately with sticky rice and crunchy vegetables.

4. Enjoy!

Savory Dutch Baby

Things To Get

for 2 servings

DUTCH BABY

- 3 large eggs, room temperature

- 1 tablespoon unsalted butter, melted

- ¾ cup whole milk(180 mL), warm

- ¾ cup all-purpose flour(95 g)

- 1 teaspoon kosher salt

- 2 tablespoons fresh thyme leaf

- 2 tablespoons fresh chives, thinly sliced

- 2 tablespoons unsalted butter

FILLING

- 5 oz pancetta(140 g), diced

- 1 shallot, medium, thinly sliced

- 1 teaspoon garlic, minced

- 1 medium sweet potato, diced

- ¾ teaspoon kosher salt, plus more to taste

- ½ bunch lacinato kale, stemmed, chopped into 1/2 in strips

ASSEMBLY

- ¾ cup shredded smoked gouda cheese(75 g)

- 2 eggs, sunny-side

- fresh chive, thinly sliced

- freshly ground black pepper

Method

1. Add the eggs, melted butter, milk, flour, and salt to a blender and blend on medium speed until frothy. Stir in the thyme and chives. Let the batter rest for 30 minutes.

2. Preheat the oven to 400°F (200°C). Place a 10-inch (25 cm) cast iron skillet in the oven to warm while it preheats.

3. Carefully remove the hot pan from the oven and melt the butter in the pan, swirling to coat

evenly. Pour the batter into the hot pan and quickly return to the oven.

4. Bake for 25-30 minutes, until the Dutch baby is golden brown and has risen up the sides of the pan considerably.

5. While the Dutch baby bakes, make the filling: Add the pancetta to a cold, large, high-walled skillet. Turn the heat to medium and begin rendering the fat from the pancetta, stirring occasionally, 6–8 minutes. When the pancetta is crisp, remove from the pan with a slotted spoon and set aside, leaving the rendered fat behind.

6. Add the shallot to the pan and sauté for 1–2 minutes, until beginning to soften. Add the garlic and sauté until fragrant, about 1 minute.

7. Add the sweet potato to the pan and season with ½ teaspoon of salt. Cook for 8–10 minutes, stirring occasionally, until the sweet potato is golden brown and tender.

8. Add the kale and cook for 1–2 minutes, until just wilted. Season with the remaining ¼ teaspoon of salt, plus more to taste. Remove the pan from the heat and set aside.

9. Assemble the Dutch baby. Once the Dutch baby is finished baking, remove from the oven and immediately sprinkle all over with the shredded Gouda. Top with the sweet potato and kale hash, reserved pancetta, and sunny-side up eggs. Garnish with chives and pepper.

10. Enjoy!

Power Protein Brownies

Things To Get

for 12 servings

• 3 bananas, very riped, chopped

• 15 oz black beans(425 g), rinsed and drained

• ½ cup dark cocoa powder(60 g)

• ⅔ cup almond butter(160 g), or nut butter of choice

• 1 cup almond flour(95 g)

• ¼ teaspoon kosher salt

• 1 teaspoon baking powder

• 1 tablespoon pure vanilla extract

• ¼ cup dark chocolate chips(40 g)

Method

1. Preheat the oven to 350°F (180°C). Grease and line a 8-inch (20 cm) square baking dish with parchment paper.

2. In a food processor, combine the bananas, black beans, cocoa powder, almond butter, almond flour, salt, baking powder, and vanilla. Pulse until smooth.

3. Pour the batter into the prepared baking dish. Sprinkle the dark chocolate chips over the top.

4. Bake for 25 minutes, or until the brownies are set.

5. Let cool, then slice into 12 pieces. Enjoy the brownies immediately, or store in the fridge for 1 week or in the freezer for up to 1 month.

6. Enjoy

Lasagna Party Ring

Things To Get

for 10 servings

• 18 lasagna noodles, cooked

• 3 tablespoons canola oil, plus more for greasing

• ½ onion, diced

• 4 cloves garlic, minced

• ¾ lb 80% lean ground beef(340 g)

• ¾ lb ground sweet italian sausage(340 g)

• 1 teaspoon salt

• 1 teaspoon black pepper

• 28 oz crushed tomato(795 g)

• 15 oz ricotta cheese(425 g)

- ½ cup shredded parmesan cheese(55 g), plus more for serving

- ¼ cup fresh basil(10 g), chopped, plus more for serving

- 1 egg

- 2 cups shredded mozzarella cheese(200 g)

- ½ cup marinara sauce(115 g), for serving

- nonstick cooking spray

Method

1. Boil the lasagna noodles in a large pot of salted water until al dente, or 2 minutes shy of the package directions. Drain and lay the cooked noodles on an oiled baking sheet, oiling any overlapping noodles to prevent sticking.

2. Preheat the oven to 375°F (190°C).

3. In a large pot over high heat, add the canola oil, onion, and garlic, and cook until they begin to brown, stirring occasionally, 2-3 minutes. Add the beef, sausage, salt, and pepper and cook, breaking up the meat as you stir, until all of the moisture has evaporated and the meat is starting to brown on the edges, 4-5 minutes. Add the tomato sauce, then reduce the heat to low, and simmer until the sauce becomes extremely thick, almost paste-like, stirring occasionally, 10-15 minutes. Remove from the heat.

4. In a medium bowl, combine the ricotta, Parmesan, basil, and egg and mix until smooth. Set aside.

5. Slice 6 of the lasagna noodles in half. These will serve as the layers in between the meat and the cheese mixture.

6. Spray a bundt pan with nonstick cooking spray, then lay 12 noodles into the bottom of the pan, fanning them out in an overlapping pattern. One end of the noodles should run up the center of the pan, and the other end of the noodles should hang over the sides.

7. Sprinkle half of the mozzarella into the bottom of the pan on top of the noodles. This will help bind the noodles together when cooked. Spread half of the meat mixture evenly in a ring over the top of the mozzarella, then lay half of the cut noodle pieces over the top to create a noodle layer. Spread all of the ricotta mixture over the noodles in an even ring, then

layer with the rest of the noodles and the rest of the meat sauce.

8. Fold the edges of the lasagna noodles hanging over the sides of the pan back towards the center, creating another overlapping pattern. Sprinkle the rest of the mozzarella evenly on top.

9. Bake for about 45 minutes, or until the cheese is a deep golden brown.

10. Cool for about an hour, then carefully invert the ring onto a cutting board. Slice the ring, then top with any extra Parmesan and basil. Place a small bowl filled with marinara in the center of the ring for dipping, and serve.

11. Enjoy!

Beef Cutlet-Stuffed Garlic Bread

Things To Get

for 3 servings

- ¼ lb top round steak(115 g), flattened

- 1 teaspoon salt

- ½ teaspoon pepper

- 2 eggs

- 1 cup breadcrumb(115 g)

- oil, for frying

- 1 baguette

- ½ cup refried black bean(120 g), optional

- 8 slices mozzarella cheese

- ½ avocado, sliced into 4 strips

- 6 tablespoons butter, melted

- 3 cloves garlic, chopped

- 2 tablespoons fresh parsley, chopped

- 3 tablespoons grated parmesan cheese

Method

1. Preheat oven to 350°F (180°C).

2. Sprinkle the salt and pepper evenly over both sides of the beef.

3. Cut the beef into 1-inch (2 ½ cm) strips.

4. Dredge the beef in the egg, then roll it in the bread crumbs, pressing as many bread crumbs into the beef as possible. Repeat with the remaining strips of beef.

5. Heat oil in a pan over medium-high heat.

6. Pan fry the breaded beef strips until golden brown on both sides. Remove and drain.

7. Cut the baguette into 4-inch (10 cm) long pieces.

8. Hollow out the insides of each baguette piece.

9. Spread the beans evenly inside the baguette pieces (optional).

10. Place one mozzarella slice on top of the other with a 1-inch (2 ½ cm) overlap.

11. Put the breaded beef strip in the middle, then top with a slice of avocado.

12. Wrap the cheese tightly around the beef and avocado, then push it inside the hollowed out baguette piece.

13. Slice the stuffed baguette piece into 1-inch (2 ½ cm) slices.

14. Place the baguette slices side by side on a baking sheet lined with foil.

15. Mix the butter with the garlic, parsley, and parmesan.

16. Brush the garlic butter mixture evenly on top of the baguette slices.

17. Wrap the foil around the bread, then bake for 20 minutes, until cheese is melted and the garlic on top is golden brown.

18. Nutrition Calories: 2567 Fat: 223 grams Carbs: 103 grams Fiber: 8 grams Sugars: 9 grams Protein: 44 grams

19. Enjoy!

Loaded Vegetarian Nachos

Things To Get

for 6 servings

- 1 cup lentils(200 g), rinsed

- 2 cups vegetable broth(480 mL)

- 1 teaspoon salt

- ½ teaspoon pepper

- 2 teaspoons chili powder

- 2 teaspoons cumin

- 1 teaspoon garlic powder

- 1 teaspoon dried oregano

- 15 oz corn(425 g), 1 can, drained and rinsed

- 15 oz black beans(425 g), 1 can, drained and rinsed

- 1 lb tortilla chips(455 g)

- 1 ½ cups shredded mexican cheese blend(150 g)

- 1 cup shredded lettuce(75 g)

- 1 cup tomato(200 g), diced

- ½ cup red onion(75 g), chopped

- 2 jalapeñoes, sliced

- ⅓ cup fresh cilantro(15 g), chopped

Method

1. Preheat oven to 350°F (175°C).

2. In a large pot, over medium-high heat, bring lentils, broth, salt, pepper, chili powder, cumin, garlic powder, and oregano to a boil. Once boiling, reduce to a simmer, cover and cook for 35 minutes.

3. Once cooked, mix in the corn and black beans.

4. On a baking sheet, place a layer of tortilla chips, followed by the lentil mixture and cheese.

5. Add another layer of tortilla chips, lentils, and cheese.

6. Bake for 8-10 minutes, or until the cheese has melted.

7. Top with lettuce, tomatoes, red onion, jalapeños, and guacamole, and cilantro.

8. Enjoy!

Bacon Green Bean Twists

Things To Get

for 2 servings

- 1 sheet puff pastry

- ½ lb bacon(225 g)

- ½ lb green beans(225 g), trimmed

- 1 egg, beaten

- salt, to taste

- pepper, to taste

Method

1. Preheat the oven to 400°F (200°C).

2. Cut one sheet of puff pastry into long ½ inch (1 ¼ cm) wide strips and set aside.

3. Cut strips of bacon in half lengthwise and set aside.

4. Take a trimmed green bean and carefully wrap it with bacon and the puff pastry to completely cover the bean.

5. Place the tightly wrapped beans on a parchment paper-lined sheet pan. Brush the wrapped beans with the egg wash, and season with salt and pepper.

6. Bake in the oven for 20 minutes, or until bacon is crispy and the puff pastry is golden brown.

7. Serve the twists warm or at room temperature.

8. Enjoy!

Chipotle Chicken Lettuce Cups

Things To Get

for 4 servings

- 2 boneless, skinless chicken breasts

- 2 teaspoons salt, plus more to taste

- 2 teaspoons black peppercorn

- ½ medium white onion, halved

- 4 cloves garlic, whole

- 2 bay leaves

- 6 cups water(1.4 L)

- 1 tablespoon oil

- 1 cup yellow corn(175 g)

- ½ red bell pepper, diced

- 2 chipotle peppers, minced

- 3 tablespoons lime juice

- 4 large leaves romaine lettuce, for serving

- ¼ cup fresh cilantro(10 g), chopped

Method

1. Place the chicken breasts, 2 teaspoons of salt, peppercorns, onion, whole garlic cloves, bay leaves, and water in a large pot.

2. Cover the pot and bring to a simmer over medium heat.

3. Once the water is simmering, cook for 10 minutes, until the chicken registers 165°F (74°C) when pierced with an instant-read thermometer.

4. Transfer the chicken to a cutting board and discard the cooking liquid. Using 2 forks, pull the chicken apart until shredded.

5. In a large nonstick pan, heat the oil over medium-high heat until shimmering.

6. Add the corn, bell pepper, and a pinch of salt and sauté until the vegetables have softened, about 2 minutes.

7. Add the chipotle peppers and sauté until fragrant, about 30 seconds.

8. Add the shredded chicken and mix until everything is well incorporated.

9. Add the lime juice and mix to incorporate.

10. Remove the pan from the heat and let the chicken cool for 5 minutes before spooning into the lettuce leaves.

11. Top with a sprinkle of chopped cilantro.

12. Enjoy!

RECIPES FOR SNACKS ON A CELIAC DIET

Garlic Parmesan

Things To Get

for 4 servings

- 2 cups almond flour(190 g)

- 1 teaspoon salt

- ½ teaspoon pepper

- 1 teaspoon garlic powder

- ¼ cup grated parmesan cheese(30 g)

- 2 tablespoons avocado oil, or olive oil

- 3 tablespoons ice water

Method

1. Preheat the oven to 350°F (180°C).

2. Combine the almond flour, salt, pepper, garlic powder, and Parmesan in a large bowl.

3. Add the avocado oil and mix thoroughly with a fork.

4. Add the ice water, 1 tablespoon at a time, and mix thoroughly, until small clumps form and the dough holds together when squeezed.

5. Form the dough into a round, flattening the top and bottom as evenly as possible.

6. Place the dough on a sheet of parchment paper and add another piece of parchment on top. Roll out the dough as evenly as possible, to between ¼- and ⅛-inch (6- and 3-mm) thick.

7. Remove the top layer of parchment paper and place on a baking sheet. You may need to press the edges of the dough to form an even rectangle.

8. Using a cookie cutter or pizza cutter, slice the dough to desired size. If using a cookie cutter, re-roll the excess dough and cut out more crackers.

9. If desired, use the blunt end of a skewer to poke holes in each of the crackers.

10. Carefully place the crackers on the baking sheet. If the dough is too warm, the crackers will break as you attempt to transfer them. Chill in the freezer for 10 minutes before proceeding if this happens.

11. Bake for 15-20 minutes, flipping halfway, until golden brown.

12. Let the crackers cool completely and serve as desired. Store up to 1 week at room temperature in an airtight container.

13. Enjoy!

Saltwater Taffy

Things To Get

for 35 pieces

- 1 cup sugar(200 g)

- 1 tablespoon cornstarch

- 1 tablespoon unsalted butter

- ⅔ cup light corn syrup(145 g)

- 1 teaspoon salt

- ½ cup water(120 mL)

- 1 teaspoon vanilla extract

- ½ teaspoon flavored extract, of your choice

- 2 drops food coloring, coloring of your choice

Method

1. Add the sugar to a large pot fitted with a candy thermometer. Sift in the cornstarch and whisk into the sugar until well-combined. Add the butter, corn syrup, salt, water, vanilla, and flavor extract of choice to the pot. Whisk to combine, then turn the heat to medium and cook until the mixture reaches 250°F (120°C).

2. Add the food coloring and stir to combine.

3. Pour the candy into a greased heatproof dish and cool until you are able to handle it, 5-10 minutes.

4. Stretch the mixture out 12 inches (30 cm) (or further) and fold it over itself again and again for 10-15 minutes. The taffy will turn from translucent to opaque.

5. When the taffy becomes harder to pull, roll it to about a 30-inch (76-cm) long and 1-inch (2-

cm) thick log on a greased surface. Cut the log in half. Then slice the taffy into bite-size chunks.

6. Wrap each piece of taffy in a square of parchment paper and twist the ends to seal.

7. Enjoy!

Vegetable Peel Chips

Things To Get

for 4 servings

• 6 cups vegetable peels(1 kg), such as russet potatoes, beets, and sweet potatoes, loosely packed

• ¼ cup olive oil(60 mL)

- 1 teaspoon kosher salt, plus more to taste

- 1 ½ teaspoons garlic powder

- 1 teaspoon paprika

- 1 ½ teaspoons dried parsley

Method

1. Place an oven rack in the center of the oven. Preheat the oven to 400°F (200°C).

2. In a medium bowl, toss together the vegetable peels, olive oil, and salt.

3. Spread the peels in an even layer on a baking sheet.

4. Roast for 20-25 minutes, tossing halfway through, until the peels are dried and crisp, but not burnt.

5. In a small bowl, mix together the garlic powder, paprika, and dried parsley. Toss the

peel chips with the spice mixture. Season with salt to taste.

6. The veggie peel chips will keep for up to 3 days stored in a cool, dry place.

7. Enjoy!

Dairy-Free Cashew Queso

Things To Get

for 3 cups

• 2 cups water(480 mL)

• 2 medium garlic cloves

• 1 ½ cups raw cashews(225 g)

• 3 tablespoons nutritional yeast

• 1 ¼ teaspoons ground cumin

- ½ teaspoon chipotle powder

- ½ teaspoon smoked paprika

- 1 ½ teaspoons chili powder

- 1 ¼ teaspoons kosher salt, plus more to taste

- ½ cup canned diced tomatoes with green chiles(100 g)

- tortilla chip, for serving

Method

1. In a small saucepan, bring the water to a simmer over medium-high heat. Add the garlic cloves and blanch for 60 seconds. Remove the garlic, then remove the pot from the heat and reserve the hot water.

2. To a the bowl of a food processor, add the cashews, blanched garlic cloves, nutritional yeast, cumin, chipotle powder, paprika, chili

powder, and salt. Starting with 1¼ cups (300 g), add the reserved hot water. Blend on medium-high speed to combine. If the mixture looks too thick and isn't blending well, add another ¼ cup (60 ml) of hot water and continue blending. Add more hot water, 1-2 tablespoons at a time, as needed until the mixture is smooth, silky, and spreadable.

3. Transfer the queso to a serving bowl and fold in the diced tomatoes and green chiles.

4. Serve with tortilla chips.

5. Enjoy!

Carrot Roses

Things To Get

for 4 servings

• 1 lb rainbow carrot(455 g), thinly sliced, the long way

• 1 cup parmesan cheese(110 g)

• 2 tablespoons fresh parsley

• 1 teaspoon black pepper

• salt

• pepper

• olive oil

• Chopped fresh parsley, for garnish

Method

1. Preheat oven to 400°F (205°C).

2. Combine parmesan, parsley and pepper in a small bowl. Set aside.

3. In a large bowl, add the thinly sliced carrots, season with salt and pepper and microwave for 1 minute.

4. Coat muffin tin lightly with oil.

5. Take a slice of carrot and line the muffin tin. Repeat with more carrot slices, adding more spirals to each muffin tin until you don't have room for more.

6. Push the parmesan mix between each spiral, this will help the carrots stick together during roasting.

7. Roast 20-25 minutes.

8. Once done, carefully remove from the muffin tin. Serve garnished with chopped parsley.

9. Enjoy!

Gluten-Free Crispy Fried Shallots

Things To Get

for 3 cups

• 4 cups canola oil(960 mL), for frying

• 4 large shallots, sliced into 1/8 in rounds

• 1 cup cornstarch(125 g), divided

• 1 cup buttermilk(240 mL)

• ½ teaspoon kosher salt, plus more to taste

Method

1. In a large high-walled skillet or large pot, heat the canola oil over medium heat until it

reaches 350°F (180°C). Set a wire rack over a baking sheet or line with paper towels and place nearby.

2. Add the shallots to a medium bowl and use your fingers to separate them into individual rings. Toss the shallots with ¼ cup (30 g) of the cornstarch until coated.

3. In a separate medium bowl, whisk together the remaining ¾ cup (95 g) cornstarch, buttermilk, and salt until completely smooth.

4. Working in ½ cup (75 g) batches, toss the shallots in the batter to coat, then lift out, letting any excess batter drip off.

5. Fry the shallots in the hot oil for 2–3 minutes, stirring occasionally, until golden brown. Transfer to the wire rack to drain and season

with more salt. Repeat with the remaining shallots. Let cool completely.

6. Store the crispy shallots in a container with a loose-fitting lid. They will keep for 2–3 days in a cool, dark place. Use to top green bean casseroles, add to soups, garnish burgers, etc.

7. Enjoy!

Quick Kale Chips

Things To Get

for 1 serving

• 1 bunch kale

• ½ teaspoon himalayan sea salt

• ½ cup olive oil(120 mL), pressed

• clover honey, drizzled

Method

1. Preheat the oven to 350°F.

2. Wash and cut a bunch of kale.

3. Separate pieces onto a cookie sheet.

4. Combine olive oil, honey and sea salt.

5. Drizzle onto kale leaves.

6. Put in the oven for 12-15 minutes.

7. Enjoy!

Nutritious Nut Balls

Things To Get

for 15 servings

- 1 ½ cups walnuts(150 g), chopped

- 1 ½ cups almond(210 g)

• 1 ½ cups cashew and dates(150 g), mixed together

• honey and sugar, to taste

Method

1. First, take the chopped nuts and put them in a bowl.

2. Next add the desired amount of honey or sugar.

3. Mix well until the mixture sticks together.

4. Make it in your favorite shape. For this recipe, we made balls/spheres.

5. Enjoy as is or with chocolate syrup!

Taiwanese Popcorn Chicken

Things To Get

for 4 servings

• 1 ½ lb boneless, skinless chicken thighs(650 g), cut into 1 (2.54 cm)

• 2 tablespoons soy sauce

• 1 tablespoon black vinegar

• 1 tablespoon shaoxing wine

• 1 tablespoon ground white pepper

• 1 tablespoon ground chinese five spice

• 2 tablespoons garlic, minced

• 2 tablespoons ginger, minced

• 2 teaspoons brown sugar

• 8 cups neutral oil(1.9 L), for frying

- 1 tablespoon smoked paprika

- 2 teaspoons coarsely ground Szechuan peppercorns

- 1 tablespoon sea salt

- 2 cups tapioca starch(250 g)

- 1 cup fresh thai basil(40 g)

FOR SERVING (OPTIONAL)

- taiwanese bubble tea

- sweet chili sauce

Method

1. In a large bowl, combine chicken thighs, soy sauce, black vinegar, Shaoxing wine, white pepper, five spice, garlic, ginger, and brown sugar until the chicken is well coated. Cover the bowl with plastic wrap and transfer to the refrigerator to marinate overnight.

2. When ready to fry, heat the oil in a medium pot over high heat until the temperature reaches 350°F (180°C). Line a baking sheet with paper towels.

3. In a small bowl, stir together the paprika, Szechuan peppercorns, and salt.

4. When the oil is nearly at temperature, add the tapioca starch to the bowl with the chicken and its marinade and toss to coat, pressing firmly so the tapioca starch sticks to the chicken.

5. Add the Thai basil to the hot oil and fry for 1–2 minutes, until crispy. Remove from the oil with a slotted spoon and transfer to the paper towel-lined baking sheet to drain.

6. Working in batches, add the chicken to the hot oil and fry for 5 minutes, or until golden

brown. Transfer to the paper towel-lined baking sheet.

7. Sprinkle the peppercorn-salt mixture generously over the fried chicken and basil. Serve with your favorite boba drink and sweet chili sauce.

8. Enjoy!

Melon Ball Salad

Things To Get

for 3 servings

• ¼ cup castor sugar(70 g)

• ⅓ cup water(90 mL)

• 3 whole cloves

- 1 smashed cardamom pod

- 1 lemon, sliced

- ½ watermelon, balled

- ½ honeydew melon, balled

- ½ canary melon, balled

- 7 fresh large basil leaves, chiffonaded

Method

1. First make your light sugar syrup by adding sugar and water in a pan and cook until sugar is dissolved. Then, add in your cloves, cardamom and lemon slice and boil for 5 minutes and set aside.

2. Add melon balls to a serving dish. Then, drizzle with sugar syrup and mix in basil. Let sit for 7-10 minutes to marinate.

3. Serve.

Baked Cinnamon Apple Chips

Things To Get

for 1 serving

- 1 golden delicious apple, thinly sliced

- ¼ teaspoon ground cinnamon

- 1 pinch salt

Method

1. Preheat oven to 250°F (120°C).

2. Place apple slices on a parchment paper-lined baking sheet and sprinkle with cinnamon and salt.

3. Bake for 40 minutes, until the apples are slightly browned.

4. Cool completely before serving.

5. Enjoy!

Apple Peel Chips

Things To Get

for 4 servings

- 8 large apples, washed and peeled

- 3 tablespoons sugar

- 1 teaspoon cinnamon

Method

1. Preheat the oven to 300°F (150°C).

2. Place the apple peels on a baking sheet lined with parchment paper.

3. Mix the sugar and cinnamon in a small bowl and sprinkle it over the peels.

4. Toss the peels with your hands until evenly coated with the sugar mixture.

5. Bake for about 30 minutes, tossing the peels halfway through with a pair of tongs.

6. Let cool before eating.

7. Enjoy!

Bunny-Shaped Apple Slices

Things To Get

for 6 wedges

• 1 apple

• salt water, or lemon water

Method

1. Cut the apple into 6 wedges. Remove the core and seeds.

2. To create the ears: Using a paring knife, make two intersecting slits about ¾ of the way down the skin side of each apple slice. Do not cut too deep.

3. Remove the piece of apple between the slits. Soak the apple wedges in salt water or lemon water until ready to eat.

4. Enjoy!

Crispy Spiced Chickpeas

Things To Get

for 2 cups

- 2 cups canned chickpea(400 g), drained, rinsed and dried

- 2 tablespoons olive oil

- 1 clove garlic, minced

- ¼ teaspoon red pepper flakes

- ¼ teaspoon black ground pepper

- ½ teaspoon kosher salt

Method

1. Preheat the oven to 350°F (180°C). Line a baking sheet with parchment paper.

2. Combine the chickpeas, olive oil, garlic, red pepper flakes, black pepper, and salt in a large bowl and toss to coat.

3. Transfer the chickpeas to the baking sheet and bake until golden and crisp, 40-45 minutes, shaking halfway through cooking.

4. Enjoy!

Edamame Moringa Dip

Things To Get

for 2 servings

- 2 cups shelled edamame(310 g)

- 1 teaspoon paprika

- 1 teaspoon cumin

- 1 clove garlic

- 3 tablespoons tahini

- ¼ cup lemon juice(60 mL)

- ⅓ cup water(80 mL)

- 1 teaspoon moringa powder

- salt, to taste

- 2 tablespoons olive oil

Method

1. In a food processor, combine the edamame, paprika, cumin, garlic, tahini, lemon juice, water, moringa powder, and salt and puree until smooth.

2. Drizzle the olive oil over the hummus. Serve with raw vegetables and crackers.

3. But before you enjoy, take a photo and post it on your 'gram!

4. Enjoy!

Protein-Packed Breakfast Bars

Things To Get

for 24 bars

BASE

- ¼ cup flax meal(40 g)

- ¾ cup water(180 mL)

- 6 cups rolled oats(540 g)

- 6 cups quinoa(1 kg), cooked

- 4 teaspoons baking powder

- 1 teaspoon salt

- 1 cup maple syrup(220 g)

- ½ cup refined coconut oil(120 mL), melted

- 2 teaspoons vanilla extract

- 4 ripe bananas, mashed

FILLINGS

PEANUT BUTTER CHOCOLATE CHIP

- 6 tablespoons peanut butter

- 5 tablespoons mini chocolate chips

APPLE CINNAMON

- ¾ cup gala apple(90 g), diced

- 6 tablespoons walnuts, chopped

- 1 ½ tablespoons cinnamon

- ¼ teaspoon nutmeg

CARROT CAKE

- ¾ cup carrot(30 g), grated

- 3 teaspoons cinnamon

- ¼ teaspoon nutmeg

- 3 tablespoons almond butter

MIXED BERRY

- 3 tablespoons almond butter

- ⅓ cup Strawberries(55 g), diced

- ⅓ cup raspberries(40 g)

- ⅓ cup blueberries(40 g)

- nonstick cooking spray

Method

1. Preheat the oven to 375°F (190°C).

2. To make the flax eggs, combine the flax meal and water in a small bowl and mix well. Set aside for 10 minutes to gel.

3. In a large bowl, combine the oats, quinoa, baking powder, salt, maple syrup, coconut oil, vanilla, flax eggs, and bananas, and mix until well-combined.

4. Divide the base dough equally between 4 medium bowls.

5. Add the peanut butter and chocolate chips to 1 bowl and mix until combined.

6. Add the apple, walnuts, cinnamon, and nutmeg to another bowl and mix until combined.

7. Add the carrots, cinnamon, nutmeg, and almond butter to another bowl and mix until combined.

8. Add the almond butter, strawberries, raspberries, and blueberries to the last bowl and mix until combined.

9. Grease 2 9x13-inch (23x33-cm) baking pans with nonstick spray. Transfer the bar mixtures to the pans, packing each mixture into half of a pan with a spoon or spatula.

10. Bake for 25-30 minutes, until the edges are slightly golden brown.

11. Remove the pans from the oven and let the bars cool for 20 minutes, then refrigerate for at least 30 minutes, or up to 5 days. Gently cut each flavor into 6 bars, then remove from the pans with a spatula.

12. Enjoy!

Beetroot Crisps

Things To Get

for 2 servings

• 3 bulbs beetroot

• 4 ¼ cups oil(1 L), for frying

• salt, to taste

Method

1. Start by preparing your beetroot. Wash thoroughly under water and remove the stems and root. Next, peel the beetroot and cut each bulb in half.

2. Next, slice your beetroot as thinly as you can. For ease and speed, it is useful to use a food processor with the slicing attachment; if you don't have one, just do your best to cut the beetroot as thinly as you can.

3. Take a baking tray and cover with kitchen paper. Lay out the beetroot slices in one even layer, cover with more kitchen paper, and press down. Dry the beetroot overnight. (If you can't wait this long, you can remove the kitchen paper and place the beetroot slices into an oven preheated to 210°F (100°C) for 15

minutes or until you can see the slices starting to dehydrate.)

4. Place a deep saucepan over a medium heat and fill halfway with oil. Preheat the oil to 350°F (180°C).

5. Once the oil is up to temperature, cook the beetroot in small batches for around 1 minute or until crispy.

6. Carefully remove crisps from the oil and drain onto kitchen paper. Season with salt.

7. Enjoy!

Rosemary And Olive Oil

Things To Get

for 4 servings

* 2 cups almond flour(190 g)

* 1 teaspoon salt

* ½ teaspoon pepper

* 2 tablespoons fresh rosemary, minced

* 2 tablespoons olive oil

* 3 tablespoons ice water

Method

1. Preheat the oven to 350°F (180°C).

2. In a large bowl, combine the almond flour, salt, pepper, and rosemary.

3. Add the olive oil and mix thoroughly with a fork.

4. Add the ice water, 1 tablespoon at a time, and mix thoroughly, until small clumps form and the dough holds together when squeezed.

5. Form the dough into a round, flattening the top and bottom as evenly as possible.

6. Place the dough on a sheet of parchment paper and add another piece of parchment on top. Roll out the dough as evenly as possible, to between ¼- and ⅛-inch (6- and 3-mm) thick.

7. Remove the top layer of parchment paper and place on a baking sheet. You may need to press the edges of the dough to form an even rectangle.

8. Using a cookie cutter or pizza cutter, slice the dough to desired size. If using a cookie cutter, re-roll the excess dough and cut out more crackers.

9. If desired, use the blunt end of a skewer to poke holes in each of the crackers.

10. Carefully place the crackers on the baking sheet. If the dough is too warm, the crackers will break as you attempt to transfer them. Chill in the freezer for 10 minutes before proceeding if this happens.

11. Bake for 15-20 minutes, flipping halfway, until golden brown.

12. Let the crackers cool completely and serve as desired. Store up to 1 week at room temperature in an airtight container.

13. Enjoy!

Gluten-Free Crackers

Things To Get

for 4 servings

- 2 cups almond flour(190 g)

- 1 teaspoon salt

- ½ teaspoon pepper

- 1 teaspoon garlic powder

- ¼ cup grated parmesan cheese(30 g)

- 2 tablespoons avocado oil, or olive oil

- 3 tablespoons ice water

Method

1. Preheat the oven to 350°F (180°C).

2. Combine the almond flour, salt, pepper, garlic powder, and Parmesan in a large bowl.

3. Add the avocado oil and mix thoroughly with a fork.

4. Add the ice water, 1 tablespoon at a time, and mix thoroughly, until small clumps form and the dough holds together when squeezed.

5. Form the dough into a round, flattening the top and bottom as evenly as possible.

6. Place the dough on a sheet of parchment paper and add another piece of parchment on top. Roll out the dough as evenly as possible, to between ¼- and ⅛-inch (6- and 3-mm) thick.

7. Remove the top layer of parchment paper and place on a baking sheet. You may need to press the edges of the dough to form an even rectangle.

8. Using a cookie cutter or pizza cutter, slice the dough to desired size. If using a cookie cutter, re-roll the excess dough and cut out more crackers.

9. If desired, use the blunt end of a skewer to poke holes in each of the crackers.

10. Carefully place the crackers on the baking sheet. If the dough is too warm, the crackers will break as you attempt to transfer them. Chill in the freezer for 10 minutes before proceeding if this happens.

11. Bake for 15-20 minutes, flipping halfway, until golden brown.

12. Let the crackers cool completely and serve as desired. Store up to 1 week at room temperature in an airtight container.

13. Enjoy!

Sesame Seed

Things To Get

for 4 servings

- 2 cups almond flour(190 g)

- 1 teaspoon salt

- ½ teaspoon pepper

- 1 tablespoon sesame seeds, plus more for sprinkling

- 2 tablespoons avocado oil, or olive oil

- 3 tablespoons ice water

Method

1. Preheat the oven to 350°F (180°C).

2. Combine the almond flour, salt, pepper, and sesame seeds in a large bowl.

3. Add the avocado oil and mix thoroughly with a fork.

4. Add the ice water, 1 tablespoon at a time, and mix thoroughly, until small clumps form and the dough holds together when squeezed.

5. Form the dough into a round, flattening the top and bottom as evenly as possible.

6. Place the dough on a sheet of parchment paper and add another piece of parchment on top. Roll out the dough as evenly as possible, to between ¼- and ⅛-inch (6- and 3-mm) thick.

7. Remove the top layer of parchment paper and place on a baking sheet. You may need to press the edges of the dough to form an even rectangle.

8. Using a cookie cutter or pizza cutter, slice the dough to desired size. If using a cookie cutter, re-roll the excess dough and cut out more crackers.

9. If desired, use the blunt end of a skewer to poke holes in each of the crackers.

10. Carefully place the crackers on the baking sheet. If the dough is too warm, the crackers will break as you attempt to transfer them. Chill in the freezer for 10 minutes before proceeding if this happens.

11. Bake for 15-20 minutes, flipping halfway, until golden brown.

12. Let the crackers cool completely and serve as desired. Store up to 1 week at room temperature in an airtight container.

13. Enjoy!

CHAPTER 7
FINAL CHAPTER

The journey through understanding and implementing a celiac diet has been both enlightening and empowering. We've explored the intricacies of celiac disease and gluten sensitivity, delving into the profound impact that gluten can have on those affected. From the initial challenges of identifying gluten-containing foods to the practical strategies for navigating social situations and dining out, we've equipped ourselves with the knowledge and tools necessary to thrive on a gluten-free path.

Through this exploration, we've come to appreciate the vast array of naturally gluten-free foods that form the cornerstone of a celiac-friendly diet, from vibrant fruits and vegetables to wholesome grains like quinoa and buckwheat. We've also learned to scrutinize labels with precision, ensuring that hidden sources of gluten are detected and avoided.

Moreover, we've discovered the importance of advocacy and community support in advocating for celiac awareness and fostering understanding among friends, family, and the broader society. By sharing our experiences and insights, we contribute to a more inclusive and accommodating environment for individuals with celiac disease and gluten sensitivity.

As we bid farewell to these pages, let us carry forward the lessons learned and the resilience gained on our journey toward optimal health and well-being. May our newfound wisdom serve as a beacon of hope and empowerment for others embarking on their own celiac journey. And may we continue to celebrate the joys of delicious, nourishing meals, knowing that we've embraced a lifestyle that honors our bodies and enriches our lives.

www.ingramcontent.com/pod-product-compliance
Lightning Source LLC
Chambersburg PA
CBHW061029250726
48653CB00001B/11